INTERMITTENT FASTING FOR WOMEN OVER 50

*Learn the Secrets to Delay Aging,
Accelerate Weight Loss and Reset
Your Metabolism While Increasing Energy.
Including a 28-Day Meal Plan and 100+ Recipes*

Table of Contents

Introduction

Fasting is a method of dietary restriction in which one goes without food for some time. It's an ancient ritual that has been used by many different cultures and religions, but intermittent fasting (IF) is the most popular form today. Fasting can be done for just a few days or up to several weeks, as long as you provide your body with adequate water and nutrients

Today's IF regimes are less religious and more scientific than ever before. A wide variety of eating procedures have been developed and tested, based on the belief that skipping or restricting the amount of food one eats can bring health benefits, improve cognitive abilities, or help build muscle mass. Unfortunately, not much-substantiated proof exists to prove that IF helps with any of these goals.

If you've tried dieting with little to no success, or are unhappy with your weight and health, intermittent fasting may be the answer you have been looking for. Intermittent fasting is a term used to describe various ways of reducing caloric intake, such as by not eating for some time each day. It has many benefits that can help women over 50 live healthier more fulfilling lives.

Women over 50 are among the largest and fastest-growing demographic of people who use intermittent fasting to either lose weight or maintain a healthy weight because Intermittent Fasting has shown promise as a way to lose weight over 50.

The benefits of IF are not just for those who are obese. Many studies have proven that you can still lose a significant amount of weight without giving up all the foods you love. If you're looking to shed pounds and maintain good health, Intermittent Fasting may be perfect for you.

Before trying intermittent fasting, it's important to understand what exactly it entails. Intermittent fasting is not really about skipping meals. Instead, it's more like not eating at all for certain times of the day. Specifically, you can fast a little bit every day, or fast completely for one or two days every week.

To begin your IF schedule, simply factor in some extra time each day. Determine when your meals will be during the day and set an alarm clock that will go off every day at that time. You'll be eating both breakfast and lunch at your new schedule times after your alarm goes off.

This way, your body will still be getting fed on some regular schedule instead of being starved off completely. This schedule change will help your body get used to the daily fasting cycle and make it easier to lose weight over 50 with intermittent fasting.

But here are some general guidelines for Women over 50 who are interested in trying IF:

- If you usually eat 2 meals per day, try splitting up your meal into 3 smaller meals throughout the day, with an emphasis on protein (meat, fish, and eggs) and vegetables at each meal.

- Try to eat within a certain time frame. I like to adhere to the 80:20 rule, meaning that I try to eat my solid food within half an hour or less of starting mealtime.
- Aim for 3 meals (non-consecutive) per day, and avoid eating before bedtime. Certain foods may be better consumed after a meal - for example, fresh fruit is best consumed after lunch, while veggies are best eaten with your dinner.

Intermittent Fasting, otherwise known as IF, is a way that many people maintain their healthy weight and do not gain weight during the holidays. Intermittent Fasting means that one part of the day, or meal, that individuals are "fasting." The benefits of intermittent fasting include:

- Simplifying your journey to a healthy lifestyle.
- Dramatically reducing the time and energy it takes to make changes in your life.
- Getting you in and out of the kitchen quickly with delicious recipes that you can make in just 30 minutes or less.

If you are interested in incorporating IF into your eating plan, simply take one day a week, when you are "not fasting." This could be on a Monday, Wednesday, or Friday; or a Saturday on which you do not eat between breakfast and lunch. In no time you will be able to incorporate IF into your eating plan and achieve your goals!

CHAPTER 1:

What Is Intermittent Fasting

Intermittent fasting is a way to lose weight by consuming calories during a short period. The daily intake is severely restricted, and the 24-hour fast is interrupted by periods of eating. Some people only eat from 12 noon until 8 p.m., which is called the "lean gains method" after the fitness website on which it's promoted, while others stop eating after 6 p.m.—which is generally known as "16:8."

Intermittent fasting is a nutritional scheme with food breaks lasting 16-24 hours. The second name is a sinusoidal diet, but to call such a diet a diet in the broad sense of the word will be wrong. Food breaks are not a diet, but a type of food that has become a way of life for many people. Intermittent nutrition is compared to eating because it is often used for weight loss, but this system has several advantages over traditional diets.

Any diet for weight loss will be designed for a certain period, if you adhere to a diet longer than the specified time, it will lose effectiveness, as the body will have time to get used to it and slow down the metabolism. Exceeding strict diets can be hazardous to health. After completing the diet, the weight inevitably returns; this will happen even if the calorie content of the diet after the diet does not increase. Not everyone can afford to follow a diet since many do not withstand strict food restrictions for a long time. Mono-diets are not only challenging to tolerate but also represent a health hazard; for example, popular protein diets negatively affect the kidneys.

Intermittent fasting is more beneficial than traditional diets for weight loss. This system can be adhered to for many years, while addiction and the metabolic slowdown will not occur. Nutrition will remain complete, the body will not suffer from a lack of nutrients, as is the case with mono-diets.

The intermittent power system involves several schemes to choose from, so people have the opportunity to select the type of power that suits them.

Sticking to intermittent fasting is not as difficult as it might seem at first glance. With the right choice, a suitable scheme will not require tremendous willpower and continuously struggle with hunger.

Intermittent or every other day nutrition provides all the benefits that fasting brings, first of all, it is healing and rejuvenation. In all nutritional schemes, the fasting period does not last longer than a day. This period is enough for the body to switch to internal nutrition, from a medical point of view, this is not starvation, as it occurs just 24 hours after the last meal.

Efficiency from intermittent fasting depends on the lifestyle that a person leads. In the periods between food breaks, the diet will not be limited by anything. This food system does not imply the separation of products into harmful and useful, permitted, and forbidden. Compliance with intermittent fasting does not require preliminary preparation; restrictions after refusing such nutrition are also not provided.

How Does IF Work

Intermittent fasting has been around for a long time, and different variants of the method have emerged over time. It works by balancing you're eating window with periods of fasting to regulate your blood sugar levels.

After completing a fast, most people report feeling more energized, allowing them to increase their physical activity. You'll have better insulin sensitivity and blood sugar control after doing intermittent fasting. Insulin is released in response to a variety of foods, especially carbohydrates.

Intermittent Fasting and Its Effect on Metabolism

Fasting for short periods is believed to help your metabolism.

It does not speed up your metabolism; rather, it increases the efficiency with which you burn calories. The body is forced to adjust to extreme calorie restriction during an intermittent fasting session.

To survive, it must regulate its calorie-burning by reducing hunger and increasing the breakdown of fat reserves. When you place food in front of your body, it will attempt to break it down and utilize its energy first.

How to Approach It with a Correct Mindset

When it comes to one's ultimate health and desire to achieve the targets, controlling appetite, and keeping healthy food is important. Intermittent fasting will help you accomplish this, but although certain individuals can fast with very little problem for long stretches, some people can find it a bit more challenging, particularly when they first start.

There is a set of ideas to help you out that one can use to get the best results and make the ride a little smoother.

Start the Fast After Dinner

One of the best advice one can offer is when you do regular, or weekly fasting is to begin the fast after dinner. Using this ensures you're going to be sleeping for a good portion of the fasting time. Especially when using a daily fasting method like 16:8.

Eat More Satisfying Meals

The type of food one consumes affects their willingness to both the urge to complete the fast and what you crave to eat after the fast. Too many salty and sugary foods making you hungrier and consume meals that are homey satisfying and will help you lose weight.

- Morning eggs or oats porridge
- A healthy lunch of chicken breast, baked sweet potato, and veggies.
- After the workout, drink a protein milkshake.
- Then you end the day in the evening with an equally impressive dinner.

Control Your Appetite

Without question, while fasting, hunger pangs can set in from start to end. The trick as this occurs is to curb your appetite, and with Zero-calorie beverages that help provide satiety and hold hunger at bay before it's time to break the fast, the perfect way to do this is.

Examples of food to consume are:

- Sparkling water
- Water
- Black tea
- Black coffee
- Green tea
- Herbal teas and other zero-calorie unsweetened drinks

Stay Busy

Boredom is the main threat. It is the invisible assassin who, bit by bit, creeps in to ruin the progress, breaking you down steadily and dragging you downwards. For a second, think about it. How often boredom has caused you to consume more than you can, intend to, or even know that you are.

Stick to a Routine

Start and break your fast each day at regular times. Consuming a diet weekly where you finish similar items per day. Meal prepping in advance. Planning allows things easier to adhere to the IF schedule, so you eliminate the uncertainty and second-guessing the process until you learn what works for you and commit to it every day. Follow-through is what one has to do.

Give Yourself Time to Adjust

When one first starts intermittent fasting, odds are you're going to mess up a couple of times; this is both OK and natural. It's just normal to have hunger pangs. This doesn't mean that you have to give up or that it's not going to be effective for you. Alternatively, it's a chance to learn, to ask whether or how you messed up, and take action to deter it from occurring again.

Enjoy Yourself

Let yourself enjoy the process. No one starts at the pro level, so you should go out with your friends and attend those birthday parties as well.

CHAPTER 2:

Why This Kind of Diet Can Be Helpful for Women Over 50

There are many reasons people choose to fast intermittently. Some do it for spiritual wellness and some do it to detox their body. Some adopt intermittent fasting as a way to lose weight, but this is not the primary reason for people after 50 years of age. After fifty, the internal systems change slightly and these changes cause the body to burn calories less efficiently than when you were younger. And, your body's need for sustenance changes.

The following are reasons why you should incorporate intermittent fasting after 50 into your life:

- You start to burn food and calories more efficiently. The body burns calories in the way of fat and stored food instead of burning muscle and stored fat. When we are younger, our bodies use energy from protein stores first, then move on to burning also fat stores. Once fat stores are burned, the body starts burning muscle tissue as a means of survival. After 50, the body preferentially burns calories from fat stores and after age 60, protein is not burned as a primary source of energy.

- Your body becomes more efficient at storing vitamins and nutrients. After exposure to light, the skin produces vitamin D which is stored in the fatty layer under the skin. This vitamin is essential to building strong bones and muscles. The body holds on to calcium more tightly making it less likely for you to lose bone and muscle mass.

- After 50 your hormone levels decrease drastically. Hormones are released by the endocrine system, thyroid gland, and kidneys. The decrease in these hormones causes a decrease in hunger and a general lack of energy to do much of anything. In addition to these chemical changes in the body, changes also occur in the brain which controls appetite. The brain begins to lower your need for food as it senses that food isn't necessary for survival so its signals aren't as pushy as before.

- Your brain functions better and you have more energy. Brain cells regenerate through intermittent fasting. This allows you to make better decisions and focus on the things that are important for you to do. You will find that your memory is sharper and you are more apt to be able to think outside the box as your brain becomes more flexible with its ability to create new neural pathways. Your energy increases when you fast intermittently because your body has a chance to repair itself, restore energy, and build muscle mass which can lead to less fatigue over time.

- The body returns to its natural state of healing. Our bodies in general are always in the process of repairing themselves. As we start to age, our bodies must work harder to keep the body functioning at its peak performance level. Through fasting intermittently, the body's natural healing processes increase as less energy is spent on digesting food and more energy is available for repairing itself. Your immune system powers up to fight off infections as your body thinks it's starving.
- Fitness level is improved. When you fast intermittently, you tend to find that with age, your stamina is higher and your body gets stronger. You can do resistance training or any other type of physical activity as much as you want and you won't feel tired or out of breath after the workout. Your muscles will repair themselves faster so you aren't losing aerobics-based muscle mass as much as before.
- Your metabolism improves. Many people think their metabolisms have slowed down as they age and they will never be able to lose weight or keep it off. However, research shows that a strict diet and exercise regime along with intermittent fasting can increase the metabolic rate by 5% which can help you lose weight more easily than before.
- You feel good about yourself. When you see results from fasting intermittently, you feel better about yourself on many levels.

Why Diet + Exercise Is Important

Physical activity is the third and final component of the weight-loss triad, but it is no less important. Exercising increases blood flow activates endorphins after and during workouts and can aid in calorie burn. The amount of calories you burn is determined by the form, length, and strength of the exercise. However, this is usually a small amount compared to the number of calories burned by your basal metabolic rate. The average Joe does not have the time or money to devote sufficient effort to calorie burning. Exercising, on the other hand, is beneficial in other respects. Intermittent fasting, for example, will help control your energy levels by depleting available glycogen reserves, causing your body to burn fat if it isn't already doing so. Do you recall those old-school fitness videos where everybody was all about "feeling the burn"? Exercising only burns fat in a very small percentage of cases. In reality, fat is only burned after glycogen stores have been depleted (which takes a while). The majority of student-athletes will never reach that standard of excellence. It's common knowledge that burning x number of calories (3,500, for example) equals burning one pound of fat. More precisely, you're eating 3,500 calories, which translates to a one-pound weight loss, on average.

Many people believe that working out on an empty stomach is harmful to your health. A large decrease in blood sugar levels may be one way this is real. Diabetics must be extra cautious in this situation. They should exercise as soon as possible after beginning a fast, while their body's food energy is still strong. Any type of exercise can naturally lower blood sugar levels. If someone has diabetes and can't control their blood sugar levels, they're at risk of having a dangerously low blood sugar episode. Otherwise, the body can sense a drop in blood sugar levels and react appropriately to metabolize glycogen. Those who find it difficult to exercise while fasting can choose to "cheat" by eating a small meal before working out. Protein shakes, which are rich in both carbohydrates and proteins, are notorious for this. Depending on how much powder is used, mixing whey protein with water may have anything from 120 to 400 calories. When you combine it with milk, the calorie content skyrockets. Protein shakes, on the other hand, aren't usually needed to get through exercise.

If you've become used to the fat-burning stage of a low-carb diet, the daily exercise would be easier to maintain even when you're fasting. It will be difficult to get a complete workout during the first week of Keto. Trying to exercise when fasting is also difficult because you can experience low blood sugar symptoms. Diabetics must take care to avoid them. Since diabetics should check their blood sugar levels daily, a blood-meter test should be scheduled immediately before they decide to exercise. They do not do exercise if their blood sugar is too low. They can, at the very least, eat something to restore these levels to a safe range for physical activity. If you experience any signs of increased dizziness, lightheadedness, vomiting, or loss of consciousness, you should stop working out.

The types of exercises you choose will be determined by your fitness goals. Resistance training at least twice a week, in addition to the normal 150 minutes of moderate to vigorous aerobic exercise each week, is a strong general recommendation for people who want to be healthier. To gain even more advantages, these 150 minutes can be increased to 300 minutes. These benefits include a lower risk of cardiovascular disease, a lower risk of cancer, and a higher weight-loss ability from only physical activity. Whether or not a full 300 minutes of exercise per week can be sustained while fasting depends on the person's fitness level as well as their fasting routines—for example, anyone following the "5:2" Method may simply choose not to exercise on their fasting days. Others who fast every day by missing breakfast (and fasting overnight) can plan to work out after the fast is over. It's a good idea to break the fast with a small meal before completing the exercise. Exercise becomes more difficult on longer fasts (1–3 days or more). The factors remain the same, and the probability of a low blood sugar episode rises.

CHAPTER 3:

Benefits for the Body After 50

Intermittent fasting is all the rage. Some of you might even consider it a fad. We certainly believe it has some incredible health and weight loss benefits. We talk about the pros and cons and a gentler and kinder approach to intermittent fasting. I have been coaching women for decades in the area of weight loss and health, and we are what you would consider mature women on 50. There are so many great health benefits to intermittent fasting like:

1. Improved brain function
2. Fat burning of course
3. Increased metabolism
4. Anti-aging benefits

There're so many benefits there are some downsides, especially for women in our age range, and why would you know we've mentioned at the beginning that this seems like a fad. The truth is it's healthy, and we wanted to become your new neural if you thought back 200 years ago the average woman lived on a farm. She got up at the crack of dawn and went to bed right about sunset, and she probably only ate about maybe 11 or 12 hours a day tied her first meal at 9:00 a.m. maybe stopped eating at 6 or 7 p.m.

She was naturally fasting, and she was getting some of the health benefits. Of course, the weight loss benefits shade a lot more calories. So, that what we're asking you to start with and consider is what was a healthy normal in days past Robin was mentioning there are some downsides that we want to talk about before we tell you ours.

Weight Loss in a Healthy Manner

As you know, there are many ways to lose weight. However, one of the most popular methods being used to lose weight is intermittent fasting, and there is a good reason behind it. Many people don't know this, but intermittent fasting is perhaps the best way for someone to lose "body fat" instead of "body-weight." When following most diets, followers tend to lose a ton of weight, but most of the time it is muscle and water weight they are losing.

Increased Longevity

There have been many studies showings that intermittent fasting can boost longevity. As you might know by now that fasting can help with cell rejuvenation or also known as autophagy, this process enables you to get rid of the old and weak cell and replace it with newer stronger ones. This process has been shown to increase longevity and overall well-being, which is one of the reasons why intermittent fasting can help you live a longer life.

Moreover, some studies are showing that reducing calories in animals by 30% to 40% has shown to increase their lifespan. However, there is no study done on humans claiming such. Nonetheless, some studies are suggesting that monkeys that ate less lived longer. However, there was another study indicating that it wasn't the case on a 25-year-old long study done by another party.

Prevent Diseases

There are many diseases present in today's day and age, and it very common to meet someone suffering from one. This means we need to figure out a way to reduce the risk of diseases for overall health and well-being. Intermittent has shown to lower the risk of many diseases, and we will be discussing all the diseases intermittent fasting can help get rid of. Two of the many diseases intermittent fasting could help manage are Alzheimer's and Parkinson's.

As you know, intermittent fasting helps to boost brain health and to lower the risk of neurogenic diseases. Some studies are showing that intermittent fasting can help reduce the risk of depression, even though some people might not consider this a condition, it is still a significant issue in our society. Intermittent fasting has also been shown to reduce cholesterol, a 2010 study on overweight women found that fasting improved hosts of health complications including cholesterol levels (LDL) and blood pressure which is also known as the silent killer.

Intermittent fasting also helps with reducing type 2 diabetes, and there was one study done on men, which showed that intermittent fasting helped them stop insulin treatment. Although we don't recommend, you try this if you have type 2 diabetes that goes to show you the power of intermittent fasting and insulin resistance.

Reduce Stress and Inflammation

Intermittent fasting has shown a significant reduction in inflammation. As you know, information causes a lot of many chronic diseases such as Alzheimer's, dementia, obesity, diabetes, and much more. Now, there are many ways that intermittent fasting helps you get rid of inflammation. The first one being autophagy, as you know intermittent fasting helps you with cell rejuvenation cleans up itself by eating out the old self and rejuvenating them with the newer stronger ones. If your body does not rejuvenate itself with more modern cells, the older ones that have stayed for an extended time can cause inflammation. As you know, the average diet does not allow for cell rejuvenation to happen; this is where intermittent fasting comes in as it has been proven to help with the process of autophagy. Another way intermittent fasting enables you to get rid of inflammation would be by producing ketones. When you are fasting, your body uses up all the glycogen stores, which makes it start using stored fat for fuel, and when fats are broken down for energy ketones are produced. One of the most popular ketones in your body will block a part of your immune system, which is responsible for inflammatory disorders. Another way intermittent fasting helps you lower the risk of inflammation is by making you insulin sensitive, and when your body becomes insulin resistant, you will be holding much glucose in your bloodstream. More glucose in your blood will create inflammation, and intermittent fasting allows your body to get rid of all the glucose, which helps you reduce inflammation in your body.

Body Detox and Cell Cleaned

Detoxing your body is very important when it comes to living a long healthy life, many people detox their body thru juice cleanse or other methods out there when the truth is that they don't work. Time and time again, intermittent fasting has shown to help detox your body at both the cellular level and digestive level, which means intermittent fasting is a lot more superior when it comes to cleaning your body.

As you know, from a cellular level intermittent fasting detoxifies your body with the process of autophagy, what this process does is eat out the bad cells and replace them with healthier and much stronger cells. Through this process, you will notice benefits such as a stronger immune system, prevention of diseases, and insulin sensitivity. It has also been shown to reduce the risk of cancer, which is a great thing to know. Overall, this is how intermittent fasting detoxifies your body from a cellular level. Let's talk about how intermittent fasting helps you detoxify from a digestive level standpoint.

People say that your gut is your second brain, and studies are showing how your stomach and mind are connected. This means if your digestive system isn't functioning at its utmost peak, then chances are your brain won't either. It is very important to have a gut that is clean and working correctly, and intermittent helps a lot with this process.

Improved Insulin Sensitivity

As you know, intermittent fasting helps you get more insulin sensitive, which helps you with many things. To understand it better, let me explain to you how insulin works. Every time you eat a meal, your insulin spikes up, then insulin is used to shuttle food either to muscle or your fat store.

When you have too much glycogen in your bloodstream, your body will send that energy to your fat stores. Whereas if you're insulin sensitive, your body will send the glycogen to muscle stores and will be used for energy. When you are insulin sensitive, you are more likely to use up all the glycogen from your food faster, and not requiring your glycogen to be converted into fats.

Other Advantages of Intermittent Fasting

Intermittent fasting has incredible benefits not only to women's bodies and brains but also to men. The following are a few of the benefits linked to intermittent starvation:

Lose of weight and Belly Calories: Intermittent fasting is done to lose weight as you only take in a few meals. Intermittent fasting enhances your metabolic rate, which helps your body burn excess fats such as belly fats. Studies show that intermittent fasting leads to a 3-8 percent weight loss if done for around three to twenty-four weeks. Observation shows that within this fasting duration, four to seven percent of people lost their belly fats, one of the toxic fats in a human's body responsible for various illnesses.

Reduces the Resistance of Insulin: Intermittent fasting reduces the insulin levels in your body that in turn lowers risks of Type 2 Diabetes, which has been a common illness. The common characteristics of diabetes include high levels of blood sugar in the situation of insulin battle. Thus, intermittent fasting helps in lowering the levels of insulin, which helps in preventing this illness. It also helps protect against any possible damages that can affect your kidneys.

Reduction of oxidative constant worry and body inflammation: Intermittent fasting helps reduce stress, which is one of the riskiest ways of fast aging as well as other chronic illnesses. Free radicals are the molecules responsible for reacting with molecules such as DNA and proteins and destroy them. Intermittent fasting, therefore, helps fight body inflammation and destroy any molecules responsible for constant worries.

CHAPTER 4:

False Myths About IF Diet

Issues that are not popular can be misunderstood with a lot of misconceptions and myths surrounding them. Intermittent fasting is one such issue. Many people with half-baked information suddenly become experts on the topic and are always willing to give advice to anyone willing to listen. It doesn't matter how long a false premise is considered correct, once the evidence is present, the error is exposed, and wise people will know to stick with the facts.

Myth 1: Intermittent Fasting is Unsafe for Older Adults

Anyone can engage in intermittent fasting as long as they do not have any medical conditions and are not pregnant or lactating. Of course, our bodies do not all have the same tolerance levels even in people that look exactly alike. If one or more persons respond negatively to intermittent fasting because they are advanced in age and are women, it does not mean that another will react the same way.

There is no doubt that intermittent fasting is not meant for everyone. Fasting is not safe for children because they need all the food they can get for continual development. Fasting in itself is not an issue for older people – any adult can fast.

Myth 2: You Gain Weight as You Age

A myth is a combination of facts and falsehood. This is a typical example of that. It is saying that growing older means your metabolism will slow down and your body will not burn or use up calories as fast as when you were younger. However, weight gain in older adults is not a given. The key to keeping your body performing optimally is to develop and maintain healthy habits such as fasting intermittently, drinking enough water, reducing stress levels, and getting adequate exercise.

Myth 3: Your Metabolism Slows Down During Fasting

This myth represents one of those big misunderstandings I mentioned earlier. The difference between calorie restriction and deliberately choosing when to take in calories is huge. Intermittent fasting does not necessarily limit calorie intake neither does it make you starve. It is when a person starves or under-eats that changes occur in their metabolic rate. But there is no change whatsoever in your metabolism when you delay eating for a few hours by fasting intermittently.

Myth 4: You Will Get Fat if You Skip Breakfast

"Breakfast is the most important meal of the day!" This is one of the more popular urban myths about intermittent fasting. It is in the same category with the myths, "Santa doesn't give you presents if you are naughty," and "carrots give you night vision." Some people will readily point to a relative or friend who is fat because they don't eat breakfast. But the question is: are they fat because they don't eat breakfast? Or do they skip breakfast because they are fat and want to reduce their calorie intake?

The best way to collect unbiased data when conducting scientific studies is through randomized controlled trials (RTC). After a careful study of 13 different RTCs on the relationship between weight gain and eating or skipping breakfast, researchers from Melbourne, Australia found that both overweight and normal-weight participants who ate breakfast gained more weight than participants who skipped breakfast. The researchers also found that there's a higher rate of calorie consumption later in the day in participants who ate breakfast. This puts a hole in the popular notion that skipping breakfast will make people overeat later in the day (Harvard Medical School, 2019).

The truth is, there is nothing spectacular about eating breakfast as far as weight management is concerned. There is limited scientific evidence disproving or supporting the idea that breakfast influences weight. Instead, studies only show that there is no difference in weight loss or gain when one eats or skips breakfast.

Myth 5: Exercise Is Harmful to Older Adults Especially While Fasting

No. It is not harmful to exercise while fasting. And no, exercise is not harmful to older adults, whether they are fasting or not. On the contrary, exercising during your fasting window helps to burn stored fats in the body. When you perform physical activities after eating, your body tries to burn off new calories that are ingested from your meal. But when you exercise on an empty or nearly empty stomach, your body burns fats that are stored already and keeps you fit.

What is harmful to older adults is not engaging in exercises at all. A lack of exercise or adequate physical activity in older adults is linked to diabetes, heart disease, and obesity among other health conditions.

Researchers from Harvard Medical School demonstrated in a landmark study that frail and old women could regain functional loss through resistance exercise (Harvard Medical School, 2007). For ten weeks, participants from a nursing home (100 women aged between 72 and 98) performed resistance exercises three times a week. At the end of 10 weeks, the participants could walk faster, further, climb more stairs, and lift a great deal of weight than their inactive counterparts. Also, a 10-year study of healthy aging by researchers with the MacArthur Study of Aging in America found that older adults (people between 70 and 80 years) can get physically fit whether or not they have been exercising at their younger age. The bottom line is, as long as you can move the muscles in your body, do it because it is safe and will only help you live a better and longer life.

Myth 6: Eating Frequently Reduces Hunger

There is mixed scientific evidence in this regard. Some studies show that eating frequently reduces hunger in some people. On the other hand, other studies show the exact opposite. Interestingly, at least one study shows no difference in the frequency of eating and how it influences hunger (US National Library of Medicine, 2013). Eating can help some people get over cravings and excessive hunger, but there is no shred of evidence to prove that it applies to everyone.

~ 23 ~

CHAPTER 5:

Possible Risks of Intermittent Fasting

The risks of intermittent fasting are varied. If people fast when they shouldn't, then the risks of intermittent fasting can be quite severe. However, for most people, intermittent fasting isn't very risky. The risks you'll run into are bingeing, malnutrition, and difficulty with maintaining the fast. We've talked about bingeing quite extensively, so we're not going to discuss it much more. Suffice it to say, bingeing while you fast risks any of the benefits from fasting you might originally have. A bigger risk is malnutrition.

Malnutrition sounds alarming, but for the most part, you can prevent this by having well-balanced meals during your eating windows. The risk of malnutrition comes especially during the kinds of fast which include a very-low-calorie restriction on fasting days. Fasts like this are 5:2 fasts and alternate-day fasting. If you're not eating the right nutrition throughout your week, the reduction in calories plus the poor nutrition can result in some of your dietary needs not being met. This could result in more weight loss, but also more muscle loss and other issues. To prevent this risk, you can ensure that your meals are nutritious and well-balanced. Have a variety of fruits and vegetables, try different meats and seafood, and include grains unless you're following a specific diet like the keto diet.

Associated with malnutrition is dehydration. We get a lot of our daily water intake from the food we eat. But if you're eating a reduced amount of food during your day, or no food during your day, you're going to need to drink a lot more water than you normally do. If you're not keeping track of your hydration levels, you can drink too little. To combat this risk, ensure that you're drinking enough by keeping a hydration journal. You could also track it in an app. Set up reminders to drink water and check your urine color. Light-colored urine means good hydration, so check often despite how disgusting it might be to you.

Because fasting can be difficult to start, this can be one of the risks associated with it. You're going to feel hungry during the first couple of weeks of following your fasting schedule. You may even feel uncomfortable, with mood swings, different bowel movements, and sleep disruptions. All of this can lead to you struggling with starting the fasts. They can also lead you to ignore greater warning signs that you shouldn't fast. These signs include changed heart rate, feelings of weakness, and extreme fatigue. These feelings shouldn't be ignored during the start. If you feel severely uncomfortable when you start your fast, you should stop and speak with your doctor.

Disadvantages of Intermittent Fasting

Unfortunately, intermittent fasting has cons too, especially for females. Studies show that before trying intermittent fasting, you should always contact your physician. The following are the disadvantages associated with intermittent fasting:

It Is Not Risk-Free: Intermittent fasting is not advisable to people who are at higher health risks such as those over sixty-five years. People under medical conditions, high fat needs, the diabetic, the underweight, the underage, pregnant, and those breastfeeding cannot undertake intermittent fasting.

You Will Be Hungry: During intermittent fasting, you might have a grumbling stomach, especially if you have correctly been observing the correct dietary plans. You should avoid looking at, smelling, or even thinking about food while fasting since these triggers the releasing o gastric acids in your stomach, which then makes you hungry. Engage in some other activities but if you wish to fill your water, drink herbal tea or other drinks free from calories. You may note increased food intake in the non-eating days where you are not limited to any calorie intakes. Intermittent fasting triggers binge food consumption. There could also be cases of cravings, especially after increased levels of cortisol hormone.

Dehydration: Lack of eating may make you forget to take water. You might fail to take note of the thirst cues when fasting.

Fatigue: Intermittent fasting makes you feel tired, especially if you are trying it for the first time. Your body tends to run short of energy and disrupts your sleep patterns, and this comes along with a feeling of being tired.

Irritability: Since intermittent fasting helps in mood regulation, it can as well regulate your appetite. It leads to being depressed and upset.

Intermittent Fasting Long-Term Consequences Are Not Known: Since no one knows whether after losing weight, you will maintain the same for some years, studies claim that no relevant evidence supports the extent of intermittent fasting. You are therefore always advised to talk to your doctor for sound advice on how you should practice intermittent fasting.

CHAPTER 6:

Different Types of IF diet

16:8 Method

This is just about the most popular fasting methods since it's so schedule-based, meaning there are no surprises. This will give you the freedom to control when you eat based on the everyday life of yours. The sixteen is the number of hours you're likely to be fasting, which may also be lowered to twelve or perhaps fourteen hours if that fits into your life better. Then you're eating period is going to be between eight and ten hours every day. This might seem daunting, but it just means that you are skipping an entire meal. Many people choose to begin their fast around 7 or 8 p.m. and then do not eat until 11 or noon the next day, which means they fast for the recommended 16 hours. Of course, it isn't as bad as it sounds since they are sleeping during this time, so what it comes down to is eating dinner and then not eating the next day again around lunch, so you are just skipping breakfast. You will be doing it every day, so finding the hours that work for you are important. If you work the third shift, then switching you're eating period around to fit into your schedule is important. If you find yourself being run down and sluggish, tweak your fasting hours until you find a healthy balance. Granted, there will be some adjustment because chances are, your body is not accustomed to skipping entire meals. However, this should go away after a couple of weeks, and if it doesn't, then try starting your fasting period earlier in the day, allowing you to eat earlier the next, or alter it however you need to feel healthy and happy.

Lean-Gains Method (14:10)

The lean-gains method has several different incarnations on the web, but its fame comes from the fact that it helps shed fat while building it into muscle almost immediately. Through the lean-gains method, you'll find yourself able to shift all that fat to be muscle through a rigorous practice of fasting, eating right, and exercising.

Through this method, you fast anywhere from 14 to 16 hours and spend the remaining 10 or 8 hours each day engaged in eating and exercise. As opposed to the crescendo, this method features daily fasting and eating, rather than alternated days of eating versus not. Therefore, you don't have to be quite cautious about extending the physical effort to exercise on the days you are fasting because those days when you're fasting are every day! For the lean-gaining method, start fasting only for 14 hours and work it up to 16 if you feel comfortable with it, but never forget to drink enough water and be careful about spending too much energy on exercise! Remember that you want to grow in health and potential through intermittent fasting. You'll certainly not want to lose any of that growth by forcing the process along.

20:4 Method

Stepping things up a notch from the 14:10 and 16:8 methods, the 20:4 method is a tough one to master, for it is rather unforgiving. People talk about this method of intermittent fasting as intense and highly restrictive. Still, they also say that the effects of living this method are almost unparalleled with all other tactics.

For the 20:4 method, you'll fast for 20 hours each day and squeeze all your meals, all your eating, and all your snacking into 4 hours. People who attempt 20:4 normally have two smaller meals or just one large meal and a few snacks during their 4-hour window to eat, and it is up to the individual which four hours of the day they devote to eating.

The trick for this method is to make sure you're not overeating or bingeing during those 4-hour windows to eat. It is all-too-easy to get hungry during the 20-hour fast and have that feeling then propel you into intense and unrealistic hunger or meal sizes after the fast period is over. Be careful if you try this method. If you're new to intermittent fasting, work your way up to this one gradually, and if you're working your way up already, only make the shift to 20:4 when you know you're ready. It would surely disappoint if all your progress with intermittent fasting got hijacked by one poorly thought-out goal with the 20:4 method.

Meal Skipping

Meal skipping is an extremely flexible form of intermittent fasting that can provide all of the benefits of intermittent fasting but with less strict scheduling. If you are not someone who has a typical schedule or feels like a stricter variation of the intermittent fasting diet will serve you, meal skipping is a viable alternative.

Many people who choose to use meal skipping find it a great way to listen to their bodies and follow their basic instincts. If they are not hungry, they simply don't eat that meal. Instead, they wait for the next one. Meal skipping can also help people who have time constraints and who may not always be able to get in a certain meal of the day.

It is important to realize that with meal skipping, you may not always be maintaining a 10-16-hour window of fasting. As a result, you may not get every benefit that comes from other fasting diets. However, this may be a great solution for people who want an intermittent fasting diet that feels more natural. It may also be a great idea for those looking to begin listening to their bodies more so that they can adjust to a more extreme variant of the diet with greater ease. It can be a great transitional diet for you if you are not ready to jump into one of the other fasting diets just yet.

Warrior Diet Fasting

The most extreme form of intermittent fasting is known as the Warrior Diet. This intermittent fasting cycle follows a 20-hour fasting window with a short 4-hour eating window. During that eating window, individuals are supposed only to consume raw fruits and vegetables. They can also eat one large meal. Typically, the eating window occurs at nighttime, so people can snack throughout the evening, have a large meal, and then resume fasting.

Because of the length of fasting taking place during the Warrior Diet, people should also consume a fairly hearty level of healthy fats. Doing so will give the body something to

INTERMITTENT FASTING FOR WOMEN OVER 50

consume during the fast to produce energy with. Additional carbohydrates are also used to increase energy levels; too.

People who eat the Warrior Diet tend to believe that humans are natural nocturnal eaters and that we are not meant to eat throughout the day. The belief is that eating this way follows our natural circadian rhythms, allowing our body to work optimally.

The only people who should consider doing the Warrior Diet are those who have already had success with other forms of intermittent fasting and who are used to it. Attempting to jump straight into the Warrior Diet can have serious repercussions for anyone who is not used to intermittent fasting. Even still, those who are used to it may find this particular style too extreme for them to maintain.

Eat-Stop-Eat (24 Hour) Method

This method of fasting is incredibly similar to the crescendo method. The only discernable difference is that there's no anticipation of increasing into a more intense fasting pattern with time. For the eat-stop-eat method, you decide which days you want to take off from eating, and then you run with it until you've lost that weight, and then you keep running with the lifestyle for good because you won't be able to imagine life without it.

The eat-stop-eat method involves one to two days a week being 100% oriented towards fasting, with the other five to six days concerning "business as normal." The one or two days spent fasting are then full 24-hour days spent without eating anything at all. These days, of course, water and coffee are still fine to drink, but no food items can be consumed whatsoever. Exercise is also frowned upon on those fasting days but see what your body can handle before you decide how that should all work out.

Some people might start thinking they're using the crescendo method but end up sticking with eat-stop-eat.

Alternate-Day Method

The alternate-day method is admittedly a little confusing, but the reason it could be so confusing could come, in part, from how much wiggle room it provides for the practitioner. This method is great for people who don't have a consistent schedule or any sense of one; it is incredibly forgiving for those who don't quite have everything together for themselves yet.

When it comes down to it, alternate-day intermittent fasting is really up to you. You should try to fast every other day, but it doesn't have to be that precise. Similarly, with the crescendo method, as long as you fast two to three days a week, with a break day or two in between each fasting day, you're set! Then, you'll want to eat normally for three or four days out of each week, and when you encounter a fasting day, you don't even need to completely fast!

Alternate-day fasting is a solid place to start from, especially if you work a varying schedule or still have yet to get used to a consistent one. If you want to make things more intense from this starting point, the alternate-day method can easily become the eat-stop-eat method, the crescendo method, or the 5:2 method. Essentially, this method is a great place to begin

12:12 Method

As another of the more natural ways of intermittent fasting, the 12:12 approach is well-suited to beginning practitioners. Many people live out the 12:12 method without any forethought simply because of their sleeping and eating schedule but turning 12:12 into a conscious practice can have just as many positive effects on your life as the more drastic 20:4 method claims.

According to a study conducted in the University of Alabama, for this method, in particular, you fast for 12 hours and then enter a 12-hour eating window. It's not difficult whatsoever to get three small meals and several snacks, or two big meals and a snack into your day with this method. At 12:12, the standard meal timing works just fine.

Ultimately, this method is a great one to start from, for a lot of variation can be built into this scheduling when you're ready to make things more interesting. Effortlessly and without much effort, 12:12 can become 14:10 or even 16:8, and in seemingly no time, you can find yourself trying alternate-day or crescendo methods, too. Start with what's normal for you, and this method might be exactly that!

CHAPTER 7:

How to Overcome Down Moments During Fasting

Losing weight, gaining muscle, and getting healthy are the goals of many self-conscious individuals. When someone decides to adopt a diet like intermittent fasting, they will inevitably deal with moments of down moments. Due to the lack of food intake, consumption is limited to shortened time frames. Some might feel this as a restriction in life enjoyment for the majority and decide it isn't worth their time. Nonetheless, some find intermittent fasting beneficial with weight loss and other health benefits included. This kind of dieting can be a challenge for the daily individual. This is due to the fact food intake is limited and eventually, the body will crave more. One must have great willpower to maintain their goal and not give in to those moments of down moments. Otherwise, this kind of dieting may not be right for you. Below are some tips on how to get past these moments of down moments.

Down Moment Tip #1 – Be Prepared to Get Hungry

Being prepared will allow one to be mentally ready; thus, they will know what to expect when going through the motions of intermittent fasting. Most of the time when one isn't prepared to get hungry, they tend to give up because they aren't ready for the hunger that arises. When someone is prepared, they will know what to expect and know how to solve hunger issues that may arise.

Down Moment Tip #2 – Make Food Choices Count

While one will be limited on their intake of food, it doesn't mean that the food should lack nutrients. Foods rich in fiber are important during this dieting phase because it helps with digestion and feelings of fullness. Another tip is to make sure you aren't eating junk food like chips or candy bars as snacks.

Down Moment Tip #3 – Don't Underestimate the Transitions

When starting this kind of dieting, one might think that they can maintain it without any issues. However, during the transition phase to intermittent fasting will pose the highest challenge for someone. The reason for this is because it is during this time that people are in a steep decline in their body's insulin levels causing sugar cravings. During these transitions, people must be psychologically prepared and may even get some help from friends or family members to avoid sugar cravings. Another great tip is not going grocery shopping when hungry because that may lead you to buy more than your allotted food allowed.

Down Moment Tip #4 – Don't Overdo the Caffeine

If you are one of those people who need a cup of coffee or tea in the morning to go to work, make sure not to overuse it. Just because you are fasting doesn't mean your body is craving caffeine. Caffeine can actually raise insulin levels causing a sugar crash and some down moments. Using more caffeine during these times will only make it worse. Stick to moderation with your caffeine intake if you decide to indulge at all.

Down Moment Tip #5 – Prepare for the Hiccups

It's almost impossible to avoid the hiccups while going through these moments of down moments. They will cause you to stop what you are doing and go get something to drink. It's best to prepare yourself mentally and fill up a glass of water while continuing with your daily tasks like writing an article or doing some chores so you don't feel like you have to pause everything to quench your thirst. Filling up a water bottle and taking sips throughout the day can help as well so that you never feel thirsty.

Down Moment Tip #6 – Keep Track of Your Hunger Level

Intermittent fasting can be a mental challenge for those who are not prepared. One of the ways to prepare yourself is to keep track of your hunger level. By doing this, you are no longer going by feeling alone but added it with numbers. Knowing that according to your hunger level you should make it through the day can help relieve some stress associated with intermittent fasting.

Down Moment Tip #7 – Don't Neglect Your Workouts

Giving up on working out is one thing people do when they attempt intermittent fasting for weight loss or muscle-building goals. It's important to continue with your regular workout schedule even if you're fasting.

That way you won't feel as down about not eating because you have something to look forward to. It will also burn more calories and maintain your muscle tone.

Down Moment Tip #8 – Get Help from Supplements

Although this isn't a permanent fix, supplements can help with feelings of hunger or lack of energy associated with intermittent fasting. They aren't a replacement for food but can be used in between meals. Make sure the supplement is natural and doesn't contain any artificial ingredients like caffeine which may worsen down moments due to sugar crashes. It can help to include a small meal replacement shake as well.

Down Moment Tip #9 – Keep Your Eyes Away from Food

Food is one of the biggest causes of food cravings. It is important that when you are depressed, please do not look away from food. That means no walking by a bakery, grocery store, or convenience store.

Putting yourself in this tempting environment when you know you're fasting makes it much harder to resist the foods available inside. You already have enough willpower going on without being tempted while feeling less than 100%.

Down Moment Tip #10 – Avoid Soda and Fruit Juice

Most fruit juices and sodas contain a lot of sugar which can make you feel down even worse. They also have varying levels of calories so be conscious of how much you are drinking. Even natural juices like orange juice have a lot more sugar than you might think and they're not that good to drink when fasting anyway. Stick to water and coffee if you need that caffeine fix.

CHAPTER 8:

Foods to Eat and Avoid

Food to Eat

Berries

Berries are very healthy, incredibly flavorful, and much lower in calories and sugar than you might think! Their tart sweetness can bring a smoothie to life, and they make a delicious snack on their own without any help from things like cream or sugar.

Cruciferous Vegetables

These are vegetables like cabbage, Brussels sprouts, broccoli, and cauliflower. These are beautiful additions to your diet because they're packed with vital nutrients and with fiber that your body will love and use with quickness!

Eggs

Eggs are such a great addition to your diet because they're packed to the gills with protein, you can do just about anything with them, they're easy to prepare, travel well if you hard boil them, and they can pair with just about anything. They're an excellent protein source for salads, and they're right on their own as well.

Fish

In particular, whitefish is typically very lean, but fish like salmon that have a little bit of color in them are packed with protein, fats, and oils that are great for you. They're good for brain and heart health, and there's a massive array of delicious things you can do with them.

Healthy Starches Like Individual Potatoes (with Skins!)

In particular, red potatoes are excellent to eat, even if you're trying to lose weight because your body can use those carbs for fuel, and the skins are packed with minerals that your body will enjoy. A little bit of potato here and their can-do good things for your nutrition, but they are also a great way to feel like you're getting a little more of those fun foods that you should cut back on.

Legumes

Beans, beans, the magical fruit. They're packed with protein, and the starch in them makes them stick to your ribs without making you pay for it later. They're lovely in soups, salads, and just about any other meal of the day that you're looking to fill out. By adding beans to your regimen, you might find that your meals stick with you a little bit longer and leave you feeling more satisfied than you thought possible.

Nuts

I know you've heard people talking about how a handful of almonds makes a great snack, and if you're anything like me, you've always had kind of a hard time believing it. Nuts, as it turns out, have a good deal of their healthy fats in them that your body can use to get through those rough patches and, while they were not the most satisfying snack on their own, you might consider topping your salad with them for a little bit of crunch, or pairing them with some berries to make them a little more satisfying.

Probiotics Help Boost Your Gut Health

Having a happy gut often means that your dietary success and overall health will improve!

Vegetables That Are Rich in Healthy Fats

Not to sound topical or trendy, but avocados are a great example of a vegetable packed with healthy fats. Look for vegetables with fatty acids and a higher fat content, and you will find that if you add more of those into your regimen, you will get hungry less often.

Water, Water, Water, and More Water

No matter what you decide to add to or subtract from your regimen, stay hydrated. It will help digestive health and ease, and it will keep you from feeling as slump or tired, keeping you from getting too hungry. Add electrolytes where you need to, and don't be shy about bringing a bottle with you when you go from place to place. Stay hydrated!

What to Avoid

Grains

Whole grains may have their health benefits and be full of fiber, and you can also get these nutrients elsewhere. The human diet does not require grain consumption. The truth is while grains may have some benefits, they are ridiculously high in both total and net carbohydrates, making them incompatible with the ketogenic diet.

Some people do try what is known as the targeted ketogenic diet, which is a version of the diet specifically designed for those who complete extended and strenuous workouts. With the targeted ketogenic diet, a person will consume a small serving of carb-heavy food, such as grains, for thirty to forty minutes before working out.

Starchy Vegetables and Legumes

Some vegetables are high in carbohydrates. It includes potatoes, beans, beets, corn, and more. These vegetables may have nutritional benefits, but you can get these same nutrients in low-carb vegetable alternatives.

Sugary Fruits

Most fruits contain a high sugar content, meaning that they are also high in carbohydrates. It is important to avoid most fruits. The exception is that you can enjoy berries, lemons, and limes in moderation. Some people will also enjoy a small serving of melon as a treat from time to time, but watch your portion size as it can add up quickly!

Milk and Low-Fat Dairy Products

As you can enjoy dairy products such as cheese on the ketogenic diet, you may consider trying milk. Sadly, milk is much higher in carbohydrates than cheese, with a glass of two-percent milk containing twelve carbs, half of your daily total. Instead, choose low-carb and dairy-free milk alternatives such as almond, coconut, and soy milk.

You may consider using low-fat cheeses instead of full fat to reduce the saturated fats you are consuming. The reason for this is because when the cheese is made with low-fat dairy, it naturally has a higher carbohydrate content, which will cut into your daily net carb total.

Cashews, Pistachios, and Chestnuts

While you can enjoy nuts and seeds in moderation, keep in mind that nuts contain a moderate carbohydrate level and therefore should be eaten in moderation. However, some nuts are high in carbs and thus are not fed on the ketogenic diet, including cashews, pistachios, and chestnuts.

If you want to enjoy nuts, you can fully enjoy almonds, pecans, walnuts, macadamia nuts, and other options instead of these options.

Most Natural Sweeteners

While you can undoubtedly enjoy sugar-free natural sweeteners such as stevia, monk fruit, and sugar alcohols, you should avoid natural sweeteners that contain sugar. Suffice to say, and the sugar content makes these sweeteners naturally high in carbs. But, not only that, but they will also spike your blood sugar and insulin. It means you should avoid things such as honey, agave, maple, coconut palm sugar, and dates.

Alcohol

Alcohol is not generally enjoyed on the ketogenic diet, as your body will be unable to burn off calories while your liver attempts to process alcohol. Many people also find that when they are in ketosis, they get drunk more quickly and experience more severe hangovers. Not only that, but alcohol adds unnecessary calories and carbohydrates to your diet.

The worst offenders to choose would be margaritas, piña coladas, sangrias, Bloody Mary, whiskey sours, cosmopolitans, and regular beers.

But, if you choose to drink alcohol regardless of drink in moderation and choose low-carb versions such as rum, vodka, tequila, whiskey, and gin. The next-best options would be dry wines and light beers.

CHAPTER 9:

Breakfast Recipes

1.   Blueberries Breakfast Bowl

Preparation time: 35 minutes
Cooking time: 0 minutes
Servings: 1
Ingredients:

- 1 tsp. chia seeds
- 1 cup almond milk
- ¼ cup fresh blueberries or fresh fruits
- 1 pack sweetener for taste

Directions:

1. Mix the chia seeds with almond milk. Stir periodically.
2. Place in the fridge to cool for 30 minutes, and then serve with fresh fruit. Enjoy!

Nutrition:

- Calories: 202
- Fat: 16.8g
- Protein: 10.2g
- Carbs: 9.8g
- Fiber: 5.8g

2.   Feta-Filled Tomato-Topped Oldie Omelet

Preparation time: 5 minutes
Cooking time: 6 minutes
Servings: 1
Ingredients:

- 1 tbsp. coconut oil
- 2 eggs
- 1½ tbsps. milk
- A dash of salt and pepper
- ¼ cup tomatoes, sliced into cubes
- 2 tbsps. feta cheese, crumbled

Directions:

1. Beat the eggs with pepper, salt, milk, and the remaining spices.
2. Pour the mixture into a heated pan with coconut oil.
3. Stir in the tomatoes and cheese. Cook for 6 minutes or until the cheese melts.

Nutrition:

- Calories: 335
- Fat: 28.4g
- Protein: 16.2g
- Carbs: 4.5g
- Fiber: 0.8g

3.   Carrot Breakfast Salad

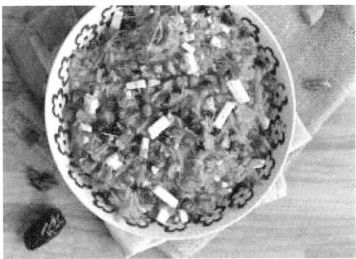

Preparation time: 5 minutes
Cooking time: 4 hours
Servings: 4
Ingredients:

- 2 tbsps. olive oil
- 2 lbs. baby carrots, peeled and halved
- 3 garlic cloves, minced
- 2 yellow onions, chopped
- ½ cup vegetable stock
- ⅓ cup tomatoes, crushed
- A pinch of salt and black pepper

Directions:

1. In your slow cooker, combine all the ingredients, cover, and cook on high for 4 hours.
2. Divide into bowls and serve for breakfast.

Nutrition:

- Calories: 437
- Protein: 2.39g
- Fat: 39.14g
- Carbs: 23.28g

4.   Paprika Lamb Chops

Preparation time: 10 minutes
Cooking time: 15 minutes
Servings: 4
Ingredients:

- 2 lamb racks, cut into chops
- Salt and pepper to taste
- 3 tbsps. paprika
- ¾ cup cumin powder
- 1 tsp. chili powder

Directions:

1. Take a bowl and add paprika, cumin, chili, salt, pepper, and stir.
2. Add lamb chops and rub the mixture
3. Heat grill over medium-temperature and add lamb chops, cook for 5 minutes
4. Flip and cook for 5 minutes more, flip again.
5. Cook for 2 minutes, flip and cook for 2 minutes more. Serve and enjoy.

Nutrition:

- Calories: 200
- Fat: 5g
- Carbs: 4g
- Protein: 8g

5. Delicious Turkey Wrap

Preparation time: 10 minutes
Cooking time: 10 minutes
Servings: 6
Ingredients:

- 1¼ lbs. of ground turkey, lean
- 4 green onions, minced
- 1 tbsp. olive oil
- 1 garlic clove, minced
- 2 tsps. chili paste
- 8 oz. water chestnut, diced
- 3 tbsps. hoisin sauce
- 2 tbsps. coconut amino
- 1 tbsp. rice vinegar
- 12 butter lettuce leaves
- ⅛ tsp. salt

Directions:

1. Take a pan and place it over medium heat, add oil, turkey, and garlic to the pan
2. Heat for 6 minutes until cooked
3. Take a bowl and transfer turkey to the bowl
4. Add onions and water chestnuts
5. Stir in hoisin sauce, coconut amino, vinegar, and chili paste
6. Toss well and transfer the mix to lettuce leaves. Serve and enjoy.

Nutrition:

- Calories: 162
- Fat: 4g
- Carbs: 7g
- Protein: 23g

6.   Bacon and Chicken Garlic Wrap

Preparation time: 15 minutes

Cooking time: 10 minutes

Servings: 4

Ingredients:

- 1 chicken fillet, cut into small cubes
- 8-9 thin slices bacon, cut to fit cubes
- 6 garlic cloves, minced

Directions:

1. Preheat your oven to 400°F
2. Line a baking tray with aluminum foil
3. Add minced garlic to a bowl and rub each chicken piece with it
4. Wrap bacon piece around each garlic chicken bite
5. Secure with toothpick
6. Transfer bites to the baking sheet, keeping a little bit of space between them
7. Bake for about 15-20 minutes until crispy. Serve and enjoy.

Nutrition:

- Calories: 260
- Fat: 19g
- Carbs: 5g
- Protein: 22g

7.   Pumpkin Pancakes

Preparation time: 10 minutes
Cooking time: 15 minutes
Servings: 6
Ingredients:

- 3 large eggs (Separate the egg whites for use)
- ⅔ cups organic oats
- 6 oz. pumpkin puree
- 1 scoop of collagen peptides
- 1 tsp. stevia powder
- ½ tsp. cinnamon
- Cooking spray

Directions:

1. Blend all the ingredients together to a smooth mixture.
2. Apply the cooking spray to the pan to coat it properly.
3. Pour a part of the batter into the pan and let it coat the pan properly
4. Wait till the edges of the pancake brown up a little bit
5. Flip it over and cook from the other side
6. You can serve it with fruits.

Nutrition:

- Calories: 70
- Carbs: 16g
- Fat: 3g
- Protein: 3g

8.   Cherry Smoothie Bowl

Preparation time: 15 minutes
Cooking time: 0 minutes
Servings: 1
Ingredients:

- ½ cup organic rolled oats
- ½ cup almond milk-unsweetened
- 1 tbsp. Chia seeds
- 1 tsp. Help seeds
- 2 tsps. almonds sliced
- 1 tbsp. almond butter
- 1 tsp. vanilla extract
- ½ cup berries-fresh
- 1 cup Cherries- Frozen
- 1 cup plain Greek yogurt

Directions:

1. Soak the organic rolled oats in half a cup of unsweetened almond milk
2. Prepare a smooth blend of soaked oats, frozen cherries, yogurt, chia seeds, almond butter, and vanilla extract. Pour the mixture into two bowls.
3. To each bowl, add the equal parts of hemp seeds, sliced almonds, and fresh cherries.

Nutrition:

- Calories: 130
- Carbs: 32g
- Fat: 0g
- Protein: 1g

9.   Kale & Sausage Omelet

Preparation time: 10 minutes
Cooking time: 10 minutes
Servings: 2
Ingredients:

- 4 eggs
- 2 cups kale, chopped
- 4 oz. sausages, sliced
- 4 tbsp. ricotta cheese
- 6 oz. roasted squash
- 2 tbsps. olive oil
- Salt and black pepper to taste
- Fresh parsley to garnish

Directions:

1. Beat eggs in a bowl, season with salt and pepper, and stir in kale and ricotta. In another bowl, mash the squash.
2. Add the squash to the egg mixture. Heat 1 tbsp. of olive oil in a pan and cook sausages for 5 minutes. Drizzle the remaining olive oil.
3. Pour the egg mixture over. Cook for 2 minutes per side. Run a spatula around the edges of the omelet, slide it onto a platter. Serve topped with parsley.

Nutrition:

- Calories: 258
- Carbs: 3.5g
- Fat: 22g
- Protein: 12g

10. Sausage Quiche with Tomatoes

Preparation time: 15 minutes
Cooking time: 10 minutes
Servings: 6
Ingredients:

- 6 eggs
- 12 oz. raw sausage rolls
- 10 cherry tomatoes, halved
- 2 tbsps. heavy cream
- 2 tbsps. Parmesan, grated
- Salt and black pepper to taste
- 2 tbsps. parsley, chopped
- 5 eggplant slices

Directions:

1. Preheat oven to 370°F. Press the sausage rolls at the bottom of a greased pie dish. Arrange the eggplant slices on top of the sausage.
2. Top with cherry tomatoes. Whisk together the eggs along with the heavy cream, Parmesan cheese, salt, and pepper.
3. Spoon the egg mixture over the sausage. Bake for about 40 minutes. Serve scattered with parsley.

Nutrition:

- Calories: 340
- Carbs: 3g
- Fat: 28g
- Protein: 1.7g

11.   Bacon & Cream Cheese Mug Muffins

Preparation time: 15 minutes
Cooking time: 15 minutes
Servings: 2
Ingredients:

- ¼ cup flax meal
- 1 egg
- 2 tbsps. heavy cream
- 2 tbsps. pesto
- ¼ cup almond flour
- ¼ tsp. baking soda
- Salt and black pepper to taste
- 2 tbsps. cream cheese
- 4 slices bacon
- ½ medium avocado, sliced

Directions:

1. Mix together flax meal, flour, and baking soda in a bowl. Add egg, heavy cream, and pesto and whisk well. Season with salt and pepper.
2. Divide the mixture between 2 ramekins. Microwave for 60-90 seconds. Let cool slightly before filling. In a nonstick skillet, cook bacon until crispy; set aside
3. Invert the muffins onto a plate and cut in half, crosswise. Assemble the sandwiches by spreading cream cheese and topping with bacon and avocado slices.

Nutrition:

- Calories: 511
- Carbs: 4.5g
- Fat: 38g
- Protein: 16g

12.   Chorizo & Cheese Omelet

Preparation time: 10 minutes
Cooking time: 10 minutes
Servings: 2
Ingredients:

- 4 eggs, beaten
- 4 oz. mozzarella, grated
- 1 tbsp. butter
- 8 thin chorizo slices
- 1 tomato, sliced
- Salt and black pepper to taste

Directions:

1. Whisk the eggs with salt and pepper. Melt butter in a skillet and cook the eggs for 30 seconds. Spread the chorizo slices over.
2. Arrange the sliced tomato and mozzarella over the chorizo. Cook for about 3 minutes. Cover the skillet and continue cooking for 3 more minutes until the omelet is completely set.
3. Run a spatula around the edges of the omelet and flip it onto a plate, folded side down. Serve.

Nutrition:

- Calories: 451
- Carbs: 3g
- Fat: 36.5g
- Protein: 30g

13. Broccoli & Red Bell Pepper Tart

Preparation time: 10 minutes
Cooking time: 7 minutes
Servings: 6
Ingredients:

- 12 eggs
- 1 ½ cups mozzarella, shredded
- 1 ½ cups almond milk
- ½ tsp. dried thyme
- Salt to taste
- 1 red bell pepper, sliced
- ½ cup broccoli, chopped
- 1 clove garlic, minced

For the Tart:

- ¾ cup almond flour
- 2 oz. cold butter
- 1 tbsp. cold water
- 2 eggs

Directions:

1. Preheat oven to 400°F. Make breadcrumbs by rubbing the butter into the almond flour and a pinch of salt in a bowl.
2. Add the cold water and 2 eggs and mix everything until dough is formed. Press it into a greased baking dish and refrigerate for 25 minutes.
3. Beat the 12 eggs with almond milk, thyme, and salt, then, stir in bell pepper, broccoli, and garlic; set aside.
4. Remove dough from the fridge and prick it with a fork. Bake for 20 minutes. Spread mozzarella cheese on the pie crust and top with egg mixture. Bake for 30 minutes until the tart is set. Slice into pieces to serve.

Nutrition:

- Calories: 290
- Carbs: 7.3g
- Fat: 18g
- Protein: 22g

14. Breakfast Hash with Bacon & Zucchini

Preparation time: 10 minutes

Cooking time: 7 minutes

Servings: 1

Ingredients:

- 1 zucchini, diced
- 4 bacon slices
- 2 eggs
- 2 tbsps. coconut oil
- ½ small onion, chopped
- 1 tbsp. chopped parsley

Directions:

1. Cook bacon in a skillet for 5 minutes, until crispy; set aside. Warm coconut oil and cook the onion for 3 minutes. Add in zucchini and cook for 10 more minutes.
2. Transfer to a plate and season with salt. Crack the eggs into the same skillet and fry. Top the zucchini mixture with bacon slices and fried eggs. Serve sprinkled with parsley.

Nutrition:

- Calories: 423
- Carbs: 6.6g
- Fat: 35g
- Protein: 17g

15. Ham & Egg Cups

Preparation time: 10 minutes
Cooking time: 6 minutes
Servings: 4
Ingredients:

- 1 cup chopped ham
- 2 tbsps. grated Parmesan
- 2 tbsps. almond flour
- 4 eggs
- ⅓ cup mayonnaise
- ¼ tsp. garlic powder
- ½ chopped onion

Directions:

1. Preheat oven to 375°F. Place onion, ham, and garlic in a food processor and pulse until ground. Stir in mayo, flour, and Parmesan.
2. Press this mixture into greased muffin cups. Bake for 5 minutes. Crack an egg into each muffin cup. Return to the oven and bake for 20 minutes until the tops are firm and eggs are cooked. Let cool a bit and serve.

Nutrition:

- Calories: 267
- Carbs: 1g
- Fat: 18g
- Protein: 13.5g

16. Herbed Buttered Eggs

Preparation time: 15 minutes
Cooking time: 6 minutes
Servings: 2
Ingredients:

- 1 tbsp. coconut oil
- 1 tbsp. butter
- 1 tsp. fresh thyme
- 4 eggs
- 2 garlic cloves, minced
- ½ cup chopped parsley
- ½ cup chopped cilantro
- ¼ tsp. cumin
- ¼ tsp. cayenne pepper
- Salt and black pepper to taste

Directions:

1. Warm coconut oil and butter in a skillet and add garlic and thyme; cook for 30 seconds. Sprinkle with parsley and cilantro
2. Carefully crack the eggs into the skillet. Lower the heat and cook for 4-6 minutes. Adjust the seasoning. When the eggs are set, turn the heat off and serve.

Nutrition:

- Calories: 321
- Carbs: 2.5g
- Fat: 21g
- Protein: 12g

17. Vegetable & Blue Cheese Egg Scramble

Preparation time: 10 minutes
Cooking time: 6 minutes
Servings: 4
Ingredients:

- 1 tbsp. butter
- 1 cup sliced white mushrooms
- 2 cloves garlic, minced
- 16 oz. blue cheese
- ½ cup spinach, sliced
- 6 fresh eggs

Directions:

1. Melt butter in a skillet over medium heat and sauté mushrooms and garlic for 5 minutes. Crumble blue cheese into the skillet and cook for 6 minutes.
2. Introduce the spinach and sauté for 5 more minutes. Crack the eggs into a bowl, whisk until well combined and creamy in color, and pour all over the spinach.
3. Use a spatula to immediately stir the eggs while cooking, until scrambled and no runnier, about 5 minutes. Serve.

Nutrition:

- Calories: 469
- Carbs: 5g
- Fat: 39g
- Protein: 25g

18.   Coconut Gruyere Biscuits

Preparation time: 10 minutes
Cooking time: 6 minutes
Servings: 4
Ingredients:

- 4 eggs
- ¼ cup butter melted
- ¼ tsp. salt
- ⅓ cup coconut flour
- ¼ cup coconut flakes
- ½ tsp. xanthan gum
- ¼ tsp. baking powder
- 2 tsps. garlic powder
- ¼ tsp. onion powder
- ½ cup grated Gruyere cheese

Directions:

1. Preheat oven to 350°F. Line a baking sheet with parchment paper. In a food processor, mix eggs, butter, and salt until smooth. Add coconut flour, coconut flakes, xanthan gum, baking, garlic, onion powder, and Gruyere cheese
2. Combine smoothly. Mold 12 balls out of the mixture and arrange them on the baking sheet at 2-inch intervals. Bake for 25 minutes or until the biscuits are golden brown.

Nutrition:

- Calories: 267
- Carbs: 5.1g
- Fat: 26g
- Protein: 12g

INTERMITTENT FASTING FOR WOMEN OVER 50

19.   Feta & Spinach Frittata with Tomatoes

Preparation time: 15 minutes

Cooking time: 6 minutes

Servings: 4

Ingredients:

- 5 oz. spinach
- 8 oz. feta cheese, crumbled
- 1-pint cherry tomatoes, halved
- 10 eggs
- 2 tbsps. olive oil
- 4 scallions, diced
- Salt and black pepper to taste

Directions:

1. Preheat oven to 350°F. Drizzle the oil in a casserole and place in the oven until heated. In a bowl, whisk eggs along with pepper and salt. Stir in spinach, feta cheese, and scallions.
2. Pour the mixture into the casserole, top with the cherry tomatoes, and place back in the oven. Bake for 25 minutes. Cut the frittata into wedges and serve with salad.

Nutrition:

- Calories: 461
- Carbs: 6g
- Fat: 35g
- Protein: 26g

20. Coconut Almond Muffins

Preparation time: 15 minutes
Cooking time: 10 minutes
Servings: 4
Ingredients:

- 2 cups almond flour
- 2 tsps. baking powder
- 8 oz. ricotta cheese, softened
- ¼ cup butter, melted
- 1 egg
- 1 cup coconut milk
- Salt to taste

Directions:

1. Preheat oven to 400°F. Grease a muffin tray with cooking spray. Mix flour, baking powder, and salt in a bowl.
2. In a separate bowl, beat ricotta cheese and butter using a hand mixer and whisk in the egg and coconut milk.
3. Fold in almond flour and spoon the batter into the muffin cups two-thirds way up. Bake for 20 minutes, remove to a wire rack to cool slightly for 5 minutes before serving.

Nutrition:

- Calories: 320
- Carbs: 6g
- Fat: 30.6g
- Protein: 4g

21. Almond Butter Shake

Preparation time: 10 minutes
Cooking time: 6 minutes
Servings: 2
Ingredients:

- 3 cups almond milk
- 3 tbsps. almond butter
- ⅛ tsp. almond extract
- 1 tsp. cinnamon
- 4 tbsp. flax meal
- 1 scoop collagen peptides
- A pinch of salt
- 15 drops stevia

Directions:

1. Add milk, butter, flax meal, almond extract, collagen, salt, and stevia to the blender.
2. Blitz until uniform and smooth. Serve into smoothie glasses, sprinkled with cinnamon.

Nutrition:

- Calories: 326
- Carbs: 6g
- Fat: 27g
- Protein: 19g

22. Raspberry Mini Tarts

Preparation time: 15 minutes
Cooking time: 6 minutes
Servings: 4
Ingredients:
For the crust:

- 6 tbsp. butter, melted
- 2 cups almond flour
- ⅓ cup xylitol
- 1 tsp. cinnamon powder

For the filling:

- 3 cups raspberries, mashed
- ½ tsp. fresh lemon juice
- ¼ cup butter, melted
- ½ tsp. cinnamon powder
- ¼ cup xylitol sweetener

Directions:

- Preheat oven to 350°F. Lightly grease 4 mini tart tins with cooking spray. In a food processor, blend butter, almond flour, xylitol, and cinnamon.
- Divide the dough between the tart tins and bake for 15 minutes. In a bowl, mix raspberries, lemon juice, butter, cinnamon, and xylitol.
- Pour filling into the crust, gently tap on a flat surface to release air bubbles, and refrigerate for 1 hour. Serve.

Nutrition:

- Calories: 435
- Carbs: 4.8g
- Fat: 29g
- Protein: 2g

23.   Morning Beef Patties with Lemon

Preparation time: 15 minutes

Cooking time: 10 minutes

Servings: 6

Ingredients:

- 6 ground beef patties
- 4 tbsp. olive oil
- 2 ripe avocados, pitted
- 2 tsps. fresh lemon juice
- 6 fresh eggs
- Red pepper flakes to garnish
- Salt and black pepper to taste

Directions:

1. In a skillet, warm oil and fry patties for 8 minutes. Remove to a plate. Spoon avocado into a bowl, mash with lemon juice, and season with salt and pepper.
2. Spread the mash on the patties. Boil 3 cups of water in a pan over high heat and reduce to simmer (don't boil). Crack an egg into a bowl and put it in the simmering water.
3. Poach for 2-3 minutes. Remove to a plate. Repeat with the remaining eggs. Top patties with eggs and sprinkle with chili flakes.

Nutrition:

- Calories: 378
- Carbs: 5g
- Fat: 23g
- Protein: 16g

24. Coconut Blini with Berry Drizzle

Preparation time: 10 minutes
Cooking time: 10 minutes
Servings: 6
Ingredients:
Pancakes:

- 1 cup cream cheese
- 1 cup coconut flour
- 1 tsp. salt
- 2 tsps. xylitol
- 1 tsp. baking soda
- 1 tsp. baking powder
- 1 ½ cups coconut milk
- 1 tsp. vanilla extract
- 6 large eggs
- ¼ cup olive oil

Blackberry Sauce:

- 3 cups fresh blackberries
- 1 lemon, juiced
- ½ cup xylitol
- ½ tsp. arrowroot starch
- A pinch of salt

Directions:

1. Put coconut flour, salt, xylitol, baking soda, and powder in a bowl and whisk to combine.
2. Add in milk, cream cheese, vanilla, eggs, and olive oil and whisk until smooth. Set a pan and pour in a small ladle of batter. Cook on one side for 2 minutes, flip, and cook for 2 minutes.
3. Transfer to a plate and repeat the cooking process until the batter is exhausted. Pour the berries and ½ cup of water into a saucepan and bring to a boil.
4. Simmer for 12 minutes. Pour in xylitol, stir, and continue cooking for 5 minutes. Stir in salt and lemon juice. Mix arrowroot starch with 1 tbsp. of water; pour the mixture into the berries. Stir and continue cooking the sauce until it thickens. Serve.

Nutrition:

- Calories: 433 Carbs: 4.9g
- Fat: 39g Protein: 8.2g

CHAPTER 10:

Lunch Recipe

25.   Cabbage Casserole

Preparation time: 15 minutes
Cooking time: 30 minutes
Servings: 2
Ingredients:

- ½ head cabbage
- 2 scallions, chopped
- 4 tbsps. unsalted butter
- 2 oz. cream cheese, softened
- ¼ cup Parmesan cheese, grated
- ¼ cup fresh cream
- ½ tsp. Dijon mustard
- 2 tbsps. fresh parsley, chopped
- Salt and ground black pepper, as required
- ½ cup onion, chopped

Directions:

1. Preheat your oven to 350°F (180°C).
2. Cut the cabbage head into half, lengthwise. Then cut into 4 equal-sized wedges.
3. In a pan of boiling water, add cabbage wedges and cook, covered for about 5 minutes. Drain well and arrange cabbage wedges into a small baking dish.
4. In a small pan, melt butter and sauté onions for about 5 minutes.
5. Add the remaining ingredients and stir to combine.
6. Remove from the heat and immediately, place the cheese mixture over cabbage wedges evenly. Bake for about 20 minutes.
7. Remove from the oven and let it cool for about 5 minutes before serving.
8. Cut into 3 equal-sized portions and serve.

Nutrition:

- Calories: 273 Fat: 24.8g
- Carbs: 9g Fiber: 3.4g Protein: 6.2g

26. Salmon With Salsa

Preparation time: 15 minutes

Cooking time: 8 minutes

Servings: 2

Ingredients:

For Salsa:

- 1 small tomato, chopped
- 2 tbsps. red onion, chopped finely
- ¼ cup fresh cilantro, chopped finely
- 1 tbsp. jalapeño pepper, seeded and minced finely
- 1 garlic clove, minced finely
- Salt and ground black pepper, as required

For Salmon:

- 4 (5 oz.) (1-inch thick) salmon fillets
- 3 tbsps. butter
- 1 tbsp. fresh rosemary leaves, chopped
- 1 tbsp. fresh lemon juice

Directions:

1. For the salsa: Add all ingredients in a bowl and gently, stir to combine. With plastic wrap, cover the bowl and refrigerate before serving.
2. For salmon: season each salmon fillet with salt and black pepper generously. In a large skillet, melt butter over medium-high. Place the salmon fillets, skins side up, and cook for about 4 minutes.
3. Carefully change the side of each salmon fillet and cook for about 4 minutes more. Stir in the rosemary and lemon juice and remove from the heat. Divide the salsa onto serving plates evenly. Place 1 salmon fillet on each plate and serve.

Nutrition:

- Calories: 481
- Fat: 37.2g
- Carbs: 11g
- Fiber: 7.6g
- Protein: 29.9g

27. Zucchini Avocado Carpaccio

Preparation time: 10 minutes
Cooking time: 0 minutes
Servings: 2
Ingredients:

- 3 cups thinly sliced zucchini
- 1 thinly sliced ripe avocado
- 1 tbsp. freshly squeezed lemon juice
- 1 tbsp. Extra-virgin olive oil
- ¼ tbsp. finely grated lemon zest
- ½ tsp. freshly ground black pepper
- 1 oz. Sliced and chopped almonds
- Sea salt to taste

Directions:

1. Mix the lemon juice with the lemon zest in a bowl.
2. Add in the olive oil along with black pepper and sea salt.
3. Thinly slice the zucchini and avocado on a plate.
4. Set the avocado and zucchini and on a plate in an overlapping manner.
5. Now drizzle the lemon juice mixture over the salad.
6. Top the salad with finely chopped almonds.

Nutrition:

- Calories: 81
- Carbs: 5g
- Fat: 6g
- Protein: 3g

INTERMITTENT FASTING FOR WOMEN OVER 50

28.   Chipotle Chicken Chowder

Preparation time: 10 minutes
Cooking time: 25 minutes
Servings: 2
Ingredients:

- 16 oz. boneless, skinless, fully cooked chicken breast meat
- 3 cups organic chicken broth
- 3 cups coconut milk - 6 tbsps. tapioca flour
- 2 tbsps. extra-virgin olive oil
- 2 tsps. ground cumin
- 7 oz. chopped green bell pepper
- 7 oz. chopped red pepper
- 7 oz. chopped white onion
- 3 chipotle peppers in adobo sauce
- 1 cup Water - Spring onions for garnishing

Directions:

1. Over medium heat, place your thick base saucepan and add extra-virgin olive oil.
2. Add the vegetables like onion and all bell peppers along with cumin. Stir the mix thoroughly so that everything gets mixed. Cook it for a couple of minutes while stirring it occasionally.
3. Add the chicken broth, water, and chipotle.
4. Always remain careful of the quantity of chipotle you add. If you don't like it too hot, be careful with the quantity.
5. Bring the contents to a boil. Reduce the heat once the mixture has come to a boil. Cover the saucepan and let it simmer for about 8-10 minutes.
6. Add the chicken breasts.
7. Prepare the tapioca flour mixture in a separate bowl.
8. To make this, take the flour in a bowl and add ⅔ cup of coconut milk. Blend the mixture properly. Ensure that there are no lumps.
9. Now, add this mixture to the broth in the saucepan and let it also come to a boil. Allow it to boil for a few minutes and then add the remaining coconut milk to the broth. Over medium heat, continue cooking the broth for a few more minutes. Keep stirring the broth at regular intervals.
10. Ensure that the soup is thick and bubbly.
11. After a few minutes, transfer the soup into a bowl and garnish it with chopped green onion.

Nutrition:

- Calories: 140 Carbs: 22g Fat: 3g Protein: 6g

29. Grilled Salmon with Avocado Salsa

Preparation time: 15 minutes
Cooking time: 25 minutes
Servings: 1
Ingredients:

- 16 oz. Salmon
- 1 Avocado-Sliced
- ½ Red Onion-Sliced
- 1 tbsp. Olive Oil
- ½ tsp. Paprika Powder
- ½ tsp. Ground Cumin
- 1/4 tsp. Chili Powder
- Fresh Cilantro- Chopped
- 4 tbsps. Lime Juice
- Salt to taste

Directions:

1. For the seasoning mix, add the chopped onions, paprika, chili powder, cumin, olive oil, and salt in a mixing bowl.
2. Coat the salmon properly with the prepared mix
3. Keep it in the refrigerator for at least 45 minutes
4. In a separate bowl, add the avocado, onion, cilantro, and lime juice, salt. Let it cool in the fridge for a while.
5. Grill the salmon from both sides.
6. Eat the salmon with avocado salsa on the side.

Nutrition:

- Calories: 232
- Carbs: 18g
- Fat: 5g
- Protein: 29g

30. Thai Tofu Curry
Preparation time: 15 minutes
Cooking time: 30 minutes
Servings: 2
Ingredients:

- 7 oz. Tofu- Small chunks
- 2 oz. Mangetout
- 2 oz. Baby corn, cut into small pieces
- 1 green chili- chopped
- 2 shallots, chopped
- 2 lime leaves - 1 aubergine
- ½ green pepper- thinly sliced
- ⅓ cup of lime juice - 1 tsp. Thai sauce
- 2 tbsps. green curry Thai paste
- 7 oz. Coconut milk
- Lime wedges for serving
- 6 oz. long-grain Basmati rice for serving
- Chopped coriander for garnishing

Directions:

1. Take a large skillet with deep sides.
2. Begin by frying the shallots on medium heat for about 5 minutes.
3. Add the salt as it would speed up the cooking.
4. Ensure that the shallots are translucent.
5. Toss in the chili and continue frying for another minute.
6. You'll see the color of the shallots changing. It would be time to add the curry paste. Continue frying for another minute.
7. Now, add the coconut milk and the Thai sauce.
8. Let the mixture come to a boil.
9. Once the mixture has started to boil, reduce the heat and let it simmer for another 5 minutes. Add the aubergine and the lime leaves. Let it cook for another 10 minutes. After this, add tofu and green pepper to the curry.
10. Take off the lid and let it cook for 5 more minutes.
11. Finally, add the mangetout, baby corn, and lime juice.
12. In a separate vessel, cook your rice. Sprinkle coriander on the top and put the lime wedge on the side. Serve it hot with rice.

Nutrition:

- Calories: 146 Carbs: 10g Fat: 8g Protein: 10g

31. Lunch Chicken Wraps

Preparation time: 18 minutes
Cooking time: 6 hours
Servings: 6
Ingredients:

- 6 tortillas
- 3 tbsps. Caesar dressing
- 1 lb. chicken breast
- ½ cup lettuce
- 1 cup water
- 1 oz. bay leaf
- 1 tsp. salt
- 1 tsp. ground pepper
- 1 tsp. coriander
- 4 oz. Feta cheese

Directions:

1. Put the chicken breast in the slow cooker.
2. Sprinkle the meat with bay leaf, salt, ground pepper, and coriander.
3. Add water and cook the chicken breast for 6 hours on LOW.
4. Then remove the cooked chicken from the slow cooker and shred it with a fork.
5. Chop the lettuce roughly.
6. Then chop Feta cheese. Combine the chopped ingredients together and add the shredded chicken breast and Caesar dressing.
7. Mix everything together well. After this, spread the tortillas with the shredded chicken mixture and wrap them. Enjoy!

Nutrition:

- Calories: 376
- Fat: 18.5g
- Fiber: 3g
- Carbs: 29.43g
- Protein: 23g

32. Nutritious Lunch Wraps

Preparation time: 20 minutes
Cooking time: 4 hours
Servings: 5
Ingredients:

- 7 oz. ground pork
- 5 tortillas
- 1 tbsp. tomato paste
- ½ cup lettuce
- 1 tsp. ground black pepper
- 1 tsp. salt
- 1 tsp. sour cream
- 5 tbsps. water
- 4 oz. Parmesan, shredded
- 2 tomatoes

Directions:

1. Combine the ground pork with tomato paste, ground black pepper, salt, and sour cream. Transfer the meat mixture to the slow cooker and cook on HIGH for 4 hours.
2. Meanwhile, chop the lettuce roughly. Slice the tomatoes.
3. Place the sliced tomatoes in the tortillas and add the chopped lettuce and shredded Parmesan. When the ground pork is cooked, chill to room temperature.
4. Add the ground pork to the tortillas and wrap them. Enjoy!

Nutrition:

- Calories: 318
- Fat: 7g
- Fiber: 2g
- Carbs: 3.76g
- Protein: 26g

33. Stuffed Eggplants

Preparation time: 20 minutes

Cooking time: 8 hours

Servings: 4

Ingredients:

- 4 medium eggplants
- 1 cup rice, half-cooked
- ½ cup chicken stock
- 1 tsp. salt
- 1 tsp. paprika
- ½ cup fresh cilantro
- 3 tbsps. tomato sauce
- 1 tsp. olive oil

Directions:

1. Wash the eggplants carefully and remove the flesh from them.
2. Then combine the rice with salt, paprika, and tomato sauce.
3. Chop the fresh cilantro and add it to the rice mixture.
4. Then fill the prepared eggplants with the rice mixture.
5. Pour the chicken stock and olive oil into the slow cooker.
6. Add the stuffed eggplants and close the slow cooker lid.
7. Cook the dish on LOW for 8 hours. When the eggplants are done, chill them a little and serve immediately. Enjoy!

Nutrition:

- Calories: 277
- Fat: 9.1g
- Fiber: 24g
- Carbs: 51.92g
- Protein: 11g

34. Light Lunch Quiche

Preparation time: 21 minutes
Cooking time: 4 hours 25 minutes
Servings: 7
Ingredients:

- 7 oz. pie crust
- ¼ cup broccoli
- ⅓ cup sweet peas
- ¼ cup heavy cream
- 2 tbsps. flour
- 3 eggs
- 4 oz. Romano cheese, shredded
- 1 tsp. cilantro
- 1 tsp. salt
- ¼ cup spinach
- 1 tomato

Directions:

1. Cover the inside of the slow cooker bowl with parchment.
2. Put the pie crust inside and flatten it well with your fingertips.
3. Chop the broccoli and combine it with sweet peas. Combine the heavy cream, flour, cilantro, and salt together. Stir the liquid until smooth.
4. Then beat the eggs into the heavy cream liquid and mix it with a hand mixer. When you get a smooth mix, combine it with broccoli.
5. Chop the spinach and add it to the mix. Chop the tomato and add it to the mix too. Pour the prepared mixture into the pie crust slowly.
6. Close the slow cooker lid and cook the quiche for 4 hours on HIGH.
7. After 4 hours, sprinkle the quiche surface with the shredded cheese and cook the dish for 25 minutes more. Serve the prepared quiche! Enjoy!

Nutrition:

- Calories: 287
- Fat: 18.8g
- Fiber: 1g
- Carbs: 17.1g
- Protein: 11g

35. Chicken Open Sandwich

Preparation time: 15 minutes
Cooking time: 8 hours
Servings: 4
Ingredients:

- 7 oz. chicken fillet
- 1 tsp. cayenne pepper
- 5 oz. mashed potato, cooked
- 6 tbsps. chicken gravy
- 4 slices French bread, toasted
- 2 tsps. mayo
- 1 cup water

Directions:

1. Put the chicken fillet in the slow cooker and sprinkle it with cayenne pepper.
2. Add water and chicken gravy. Close the slow cooker lid and cook the chicken for 8 hours on LOW. Then combine the mashed potato with the mayo sauce.
3. Spread toasted French bread with the mashed potato mixture.
4. When the chicken is cooked, cut it into strips and combine it with the remaining gravy from the slow cooker.
5. Place the chicken strips over the mashed potato. Enjoy the open sandwich warm!

Nutrition:

- Calories: 314
- Fat: 9.7g
- Fiber: 3g
- Carbs: 45.01g
- Protein: 12g

36. Onion Lunch Muffins

Preparation time: 15 minutes
Cooking time: 8 hours
Servings: 7
Ingredients:

- 1 egg
- 5 tbsps. butter, melted
- 1 cup flour
- ½ cup milk
- 1 tsp. baking soda
- 1 cup onion, chopped
- 1 tsp. cilantro
- ½ tsp. sage
- 1 tsp. apple cider vinegar
- 2 cup water
- 1 tbsp. chives
- 1 tsp. olive oil

Directions:

1. Beat the egg in the bowl and add melted butter.
2. Add the flour, baking soda, chopped onion, milk, sage, apple cider vinegar, cilantro, and chives. Knead into a dough.
3. After this, spray a muffin form with the olive oil inside. Fill the ½ part of every muffin form and place them in the glass jars.
4. After this, pour water into the slow cooker vessel.
5. Place the glass jars with muffins in the slow cooker and close the lid.
6. Cook the muffins for 8 hours on LOW.
7. Check if the muffins are cooked with the help of the toothpick and remove them from the slow cooker. Enjoy the dish warm!

Nutrition:

- Calories: 180
- Fat: 11g
- Fiber: 1g
- Carbs: 16.28g
- Protein: 4g

CHAPTER 11:

Dinner Recipes

37. Artichoke Petals Bites

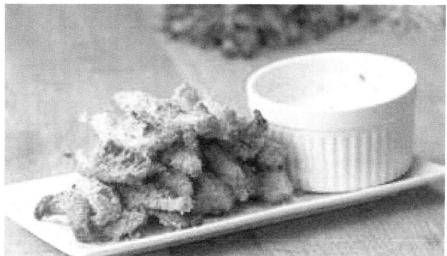

Preparation time: 10 minutes
Cooking time: 10 minutes
Servings: 8
Ingredients:

- 8 oz. artichoke petals, boiled, drained, without salt
- ½ cup almond flour - 4 oz. Parmesan, grated
- 2 tbsps. almond butter, melted

Directions:

1. In the mixing bowl, mix up together almond flour and grated Parmesan.
2. Preheat the oven to 355°F.
3. Dip the artichoke petals in the almond butter and then coat in the almond flour mixture. Place them in the tray.
4. Transfer the tray to the preheated oven and cook the petals for 10 minutes.
5. Chill the cooked petal bites a little before serving.

Nutrition:

- Calories: 196 Protein: 6.5g Carbs: 16.5g Fat: 11.6g Fiber: 2.9g

38. Vegan Fish Sticks and Tartar Sauce

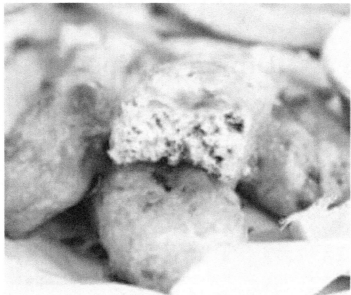

Preparation time: 5 minutes
Cooking time: 80 minutes
Servings: 6
Ingredients:
Fish Sticks:

- 12 oz. package extra-firm tofu
- ½ cup cornmeal
- 1 tbsp. garlic powder
- 1 tbsp. dried basil
- 2 tbsps. dulse flakes
- 1 tbsp. onion powder
- ½ cup whole wheat flour (rice flour is a good gluten-free option)
- 10 turns fresh black pepper
- 1 tbsp. of sea salt
- ¼ cup non-dairy milk, unsweetened
- 1 cup high-heat oil for frying

Vegan Tartar Sauce:

- ¼ cup sweet pickle relish
- ½ cup vegan mayo
- ½ tsp. sugar
- ½ tsp. lemon juice
- 5 turns fresh black pepper

Directions:

1. Rinse tofu and drain in a colander. Placing a heavy plate on tofu with a heavy item on top will help drain better. Set it aside.

2. In a medium bowl, mix the flour, cornmeal, garlic powder, basil, onion powder, dulse flakes, pepper, and salt. Whisk together. Set the mix aside.

3. Set tofu on cutting board. Cut into quarters.

4. Slice tofu into thin pieces. You should have 28-32 pieces in total.

5. In a large cast-iron skillet, heat oil on medium/low heat.

6. In a small bowl, pour non-dairy milk.

7. Dip each piece of tofu in non-dairy milk. Immediately dip in breading, coating all sides evenly. Repeat until all pieces are coated.

8. The oil will start to splatter when hot enough. At that point, add tofu pieces to the skillet. Repeat until all pieces are cooked.

9. Each side will cook for about 2-3 minutes. Watch for golden brown color. Place tofu pieces on a brown paper bag as you remove them from the pan to soak up excess oil.

10. Repeat as necessary until all tofu is cooked. Cool before serving. Mix all tartar sauce ingredients until an even and creamy sauce is made. Enjoy!

Nutrition:

- Calories: 145
- Protein: 9.6g
- Carbs: 2.3g
- Fat: 10.9g
- Fiber: 0.4g

39. Vegan Philly Cheesesteak

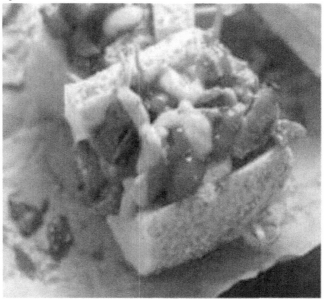

Preparation time: 5 minutes
Cooking time: 40 minutes
Servings: 4
Ingredients:

- 6-8 sliced Portobello mushrooms
- 4 cloves garlic, minced
- 1 tbsp. olive oil
- 1 whole clove garlic
- ½ tsp. black pepper
- 1 tsp. dried thyme
- ½ large diced onion
- A dash of kosher salt
- 1 tbsp. vegan Worcestershire sauce
- Hoagie rolls or another small loaf of bread of choice
- 1 cup shredded vegan cheddar cheese
- Vegan mayo (optional)

Directions:

1. Preheat the broiler. In a deep skillet, heat olive oil. Brown mushrooms in oil, about 10 min.

2. Add thyme, garlic, and pepper until evenly coated.

3. Add onion and salt. Mushrooms must be well cooked before adding salt. Cook until the onion is caramelized and softened, which should be for about 5 minutes. Add Worcestershire sauce and mix well.

4. Slice the bread lengthwise. Coat open sides of bread with olive oil or cooking spray. To add garlic flavor, cut the whole garlic clove, cut off the tip, and put on the oiled side of bread. Garlic powder is also a good substitute.

5. If desired, add optional vegan mayo. Place bread on cookie sheet. Fill loaves with mushrooms and top with shredded vegan cheddar cheese.

6. Place in broiler until cheese has melted, which should be 4-5 minutes.

Nutrition:
- Calories: 167
- Protein: 3g
- Carbs: 10.2g
- Fat: 11.8g
- Fiber: 2.6g

40. Stuffed Taco Peppers

Preparation time: 5 minutes
Cooking time: 8 hours
Servings: 6
Ingredients:

- 1 cup cauliflower rice
- 1 small red bell peppers
- 18 oz. minced pork, pasture-raised
- 1 tsp. garlic powder
- ¾ tsp. salt
- 1 tsp. red chili powder
- 1 cup shredded Monterey jack cheese and more for topping
- 2 tbsps. avocado oil
- 1 cup water

Directions:

1. Remove and discard stem from each pepper and then scoop out seeds.
2. Place meat in a large bowl, add garlic, salt, and red chili powder, and stir until combined.
3. Then stir in cauliflower rice and oil until just combine and then stir in cheese.
4. Stuff this mixture into each pepper and place them in a 4-quart slow cooker.
5. Pour water into the bottom of the slow cooker, switch it on, and shut with the lid.
6. Cook peppers for 4 hours at a high heat setting or 8 hours at a low heating setting and top peppers with more cheese in the last 10 minutes of cooking time.
7. Serve straight away.

Nutrition:

- Calories: 270
- Total Fat: 18g
- Saturated Fat: 5g
- Protein: 21g
- Carbs: 6g
- Fiber: 2g
- Sugar: 3g

41. Chipotle Barbacoa

Preparation time: 20 minutes
Cooking time: 4 hours
Servings: 9
Ingredients:

- ½ cup beef/chicken broth
- 2 chilies in adobo (with the sauce, it's about 4 tsps.)
- 1 lb. chuck roast/beef brisket
- 2 tbsps. lime juice
- 2 tbsps. apple cider vinegar
- 2 tsps. sea salt
- 2 tsps. cumin
- 1 tsp. black pepper
- 2 whole bay leaves
- ½ tsp. ground cloves (optional)

Directions:

1. Mix the chilies in the sauce, and add the broth, garlic, ground cloves, pepper, cumin, salt, vinegar, and lime juice in a blender, mixing until smooth.
2. Chop the beef into two-inch chunks and toss it in the slow cooker. Empty the puree on top. Toss in the two bay leaves.
3. Cook four to six hrs. On the high setting or eight to ten using the low setting.
4. Dispose of the bay leaves when the meat is done.
5. Shred and stir into the juices to simmer for five to ten minutes.

Nutrition:

- Calories: 242
- Carbs: 2g
- Fat: 11g
- Protein: 32g

42. Corned Beef Cabbage Rolls

Preparation time: 25 minutes
Cooking time: 6 hours
Servings: 5
Ingredients:

- ½ lb. corned beef
- 2 large savoy cabbage leaves
- ¼ cup White wine
- ¼ cup Coffee
- 1 large lemon
- 1 sliced onion
- 1 tbsp. Rendered bacon fat
- 1 tbsp. Erythritol
- 1 tbsp. Yellow mustard
- 2 tsps. Kosher salt
- 2 tsps. Worcestershire sauce
- ¼ tsp. cloves
- ¼ tsp. allspice
- 1 large bay leaf
- 1 tsp. mustard seeds
- Whole peppercorns
- ½ tsp. red pepper flakes

Directions:

1. Add the liquids, spices, and corned beef into the cooker. Cook 6 hours on the low setting.
2. Prepare a pot of boiling water.
3. When the time is up, add the leaves along with the sliced onion to the water for two to three minutes.
4. Transfer the leaves to a cold-water bath - blanching them for three to four minutes. Continue boiling the onion.
5. Use a paper towel to dry the leaves. Add the onion and beef. Roll up the cabbage leaves.
6. Drizzle with freshly squeezed lemon juice.

Nutrition:

- Calories: 481.4
- Carbs: 4.2g
- Protein: 34.87g
- Fat: 25.38g

43. Cube Steak

Preparation time: 15 minutes
Cooking time: 8 hours
Servings: 8
Ingredients:

- Cubed steaks (28 oz.)
- 1 ¾ tsp. adobo seasoning/garlic salt
- 1 can (8 oz.) tomato sauce
- 1 cup water
- Black pepper to taste
- ½ onion
- 1 small red pepper
- ⅓ cup green pitted olives
- 2 tbsps. brine

Directions:

1. Slice the peppers and onions into ¼-inch strips.
2. Sprinkle the steaks with the pepper and garlic salt as needed and place them in the cooker.
3. Fold in the peppers and onion along with the water, sauce, and olives (with the liquid/brine from the jar).
4. Close the lid. Prepare using the low-temperature setting for eight hours.

Nutrition:

- Calories: 154
- Carbs: 4g
- Protein: 23.5g
- Fat: 5.5g

44. Ragu

Preparation time: 10 minutes
Cooking time: 8 hours
Servings: 2
Ingredients:

- 4 carrot
- 1 celery rib
- 1 onion
- 1 minced garlic clove
- ½ lb. top-round lean beef
- 3 oz. diced tomatoes
- 3 oz. crushed tomatoes
- 2½ tsps. beef broth
- 1¼ tsps. Chopped fresh thyme
- 1¼ tsps. Minced fresh rosemary
- 1 bay leaf
- Pepper & Salt to taste

Directions:

1. Place the prepared celery, garlic, onion, and carrots into the slow cooker.
2. Trim away the fat and add the meat to the slow cooker. Sprinkle with salt and pepper
3. Stir in the rest of the Ingredient.
4. Prepare on the low setting for six to eight hours. Enjoy any way you choose.

Nutrition:

- Calories: 224
- Carbs: 6g
- Protein: 27g
- Fat: 9g

45. Rope Vieja

Preparation time: 15 minutes
Cooking time: 8 hours
Servings: 6
Ingredients:

- 2 lb. flank steak (remove fat)
- 1 yellow pepper
- 1 Thinly sliced onion
- 1 green pepper
- 1 bay leaf
- ¼ t. salt
- ¾ tsp. Oregano
- 1 cup Non-fat beef broth
- 2 tbsp. tomato paste
- Cooking spray

Directions:

1. Prepare the crockpot with the spray or use a liner and combine all of the fixings.
2. Stir everything together and prepare using low for eight hours.
3. Top it off with your chosen garnishes.

Nutrition:

- Calories: 257
- Carbs: 7g
- Fat: 10g
- Protein: 35g

46. Spinach Soup

Preparation time: 15 minutes
Cooking time: 6-8 hours
Servings: 4
Ingredients:

- 2 lbs. spinach
- ¼ cup cream cheese
- 1 onion, diced
- 2 cups heavy cream
- 1 garlic clove, minced
- 2 cups water
- Salt, pepper, to taste

Directions:

1. Pour water into the slow cooker. Add spinach, salt, and pepper.
2. Add cream cheese, onion, garlic, and heavy cream.
3. Close the lid and cook on Low for 6-8 hours.
4. Puree soup with blender and serve.

Nutrition:

- Calories: 322
- Fat: 28.2g
- Carbs: 10.1g
- Protein: 12.2g

47. Poached Salmon

Preparation time: 15 minutes
Cooking time: 1 hour
Servings: 4
Ingredients:

- Medium salmon fillets
- 1 cup water
- 2 tbsps. dry white wine
- 1 yellow onion, sliced
- ½ lemon, sliced
- ½ tsp. salt
- ¼ tsp. garlic powder
- ¼ tsp. dried basil

Directions:

1. Pour water and wine into a slow cooker. Heat on High for 30 minutes with the lid open.
2. Season salmon fillets with salt, garlic powder, and basil.
3. Put salmon into a slow cooker. Add onion and lemon onto salmon fillets.
4. Close the lid and cook on High for 20-30 minutes.

Nutrition:

- Calories: 273
- Fat: 21g
- Carbs: 4.2g
- Protein: 35g

CHAPTER 12:

Appetizers & Snacks

48. No-Bake Peanut Butter Pie

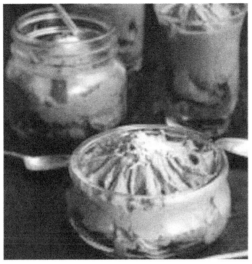

Preparation time: 5 minutes
Cooking time: 60 minutes
Servings: 6
Ingredients:

- 1 cup almond flour
- 2 tbsps. butter softened
- ½ tsp. vanilla
- 1 ½ tbsps. Lakanto Monk fruit sweetener
- 3 tbsps. cocoa powder
- 16 oz. cream cheese softened
- ¾ cup heavy cream
- 2 tsps. vanilla
- ⅔ cup swerve confectioner's sweetener
- ¾ cup peanut butter or sun butter, unsweetened

Directions:

1. Combine the almond flour, butter, ½ teaspoon of vanilla, Lakanto sweetener, and cocoa powder in a bowl with a fork until it forms a crumbly mixture. Press this mixture into a nine-inch pie plate and then allow it to chill in the fridge while you prepare the filling.
2. In a large bowl, beat together the cream cheese, peanut butter, confectioners Swerve, and remaining vanilla until light and creamy. Using a spatula scrape down the sides of the bowl before adding in the heavy cream.
3. Beat the filling some more until the heavy cream is incorporated and the mixture is once again light and creamy.
4. Pour the filling into the prepared crust and allow it to chill for two hours before serving. Slice and enjoy.

Nutrition:

- Calories: 61
- Protein: 4.5g
- Carbs: 0.7g
- Fat: 4.5g
- Fiber: 0.1g

49. Berries with Ricotta Cream

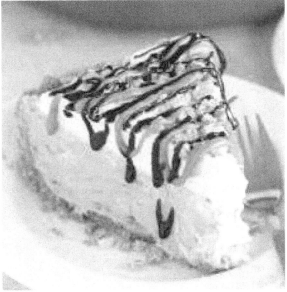

Preparation time: 5 minutes
Cooking time: 40 minutes
Servings: 6
Ingredients:

- 1½ cups ricotta, whole milk
- 2 tbsps. heavy cream
- 1½ tsps. lemon zest
- ¼ cup Swerve confectioner's sweetener
- 1 tsp. vanilla extract
- ½ cup blackberries
- ½ cup raspberries
- ½ cup blueberries

Directions:

1. In a large bowl, add all of the ingredients, except for the berries, and whip them together with a hand mixer until completely smooth.
2. Set out four parfait glasses and divide half of the berries between all of them. Top the berries with half of the ricotta mixture, the remaining half of the berries, and lastly, the second half of the ricotta mixture.
3. Serve the parfaits immediately or within the next twenty-four hours.

Nutrition:

- Calories: 153 Protein: 6.2g
- Carbs: 19.2g Fat: 5.6g Fiber: 2.6g

50. Easy Chocolate Pudding

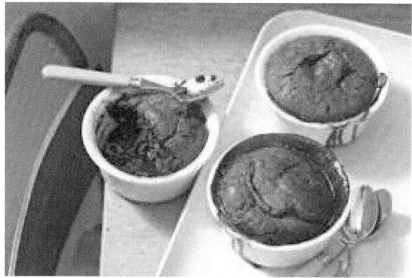

Preparation time: 5 minutes
Cooking time: 30 minutes
Servings: 6
Ingredients:

- 1½ cups organic coconut cream from a can
- ½ cup raw cacao powder (sifted unsweetened cocoa powder works as well)
- 6 tbsps. pure maple syrup (may adjust to up to 8 tbsps. depending on how sweet you like it)
- 2 tsps. pure vanilla extract
- Fine-grain sea salt.

Directions:

1. In a small saucepan over low heat, whisk coconut cream, cacao, and maple syrup until smooth. A smaller whisk my make a smoother mixture.
2. Continue to cook over low/medium for 2 minutes, or until the mixture just starts to come to a boil with small bubbles.
3. Remove from heat. Add salt and vanilla. Stir. Taste and add more maple if you'd like a sweeter pudding. Pour into individual containers/bowls or keep in one larger bowl to set.
4. Cover and refrigerate until set or overnight for a thick and creamy pudding. Makes 4 servings.

Nutrition:

- Calories: 231 Protein: 14.9g
- Carbs: 3.2g Fat: 18g Fiber: 1.1g

51. Vanilla Muffins

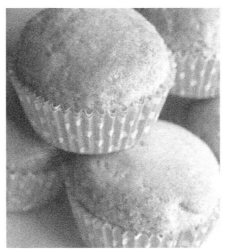

Preparation time: 5 minutes
Cooking time: 2 minutes
Servings: 4
Ingredients:

- 1 tbsp. Truvia
- 1 egg, beaten
- 4 tbsp. coconut flour
- 1 cup water, for cooking
- 1 tsp. coconut shred
- 1 tsp. vanilla extract
- ¼ tsp. baking powder

Directions:

1. Mix up together all the ingredients and stir well until you get a thick batter
2. Add water to the Ninja Foodi basket. Place the batter into the muffin molds and transfer them on the Ninja Foodi rack.
3. Lower the pressure cooker lid and set Pressure mode High pressure
4. Cook the muffins for 2 minutes. Use the quick pressure release method. Chill the muffins and serve!

Nutrition:

- Calories: 61
- Fat: 2.9g
- Carbs: 7g
- Protein: 2.5g

52. Ginger Cookies

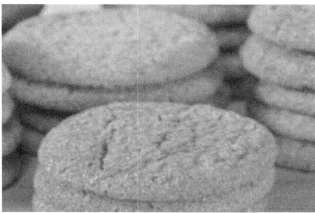

Preparation time: 10 minutes
Cooking time: 14 minutes
Servings: 7
Ingredients:

- 1 cup almond flour
- 1 egg
- 3 tbsps. Erythritol
- 3 tbsps. heavy cream
- 3 tbsps. butter
- 1 tsp. ground ginger
- ½ tsp. ground cinnamon
- ½ tsp. baking powder

Directions:

1. Beat the egg in the bowl and whisk it gently. Add baking powder, Erythritol, ground ginger, ground cinnamon, heavy cream, and flour
2. Stir gently and add butter, Knead the non-sticky dough. Roll up the dough with the help of the rolling pin and make the cookies with the help of the cutter.
3. Place the cookies in the basket in one layer and close the lid. Set the Bake mode and cook the cookies for 14 minutes at 350°F
4. When the cookies are cooked; let them chill well and serve!

Nutrition:

- Calories: 172
- Fat: 15.6g
- Carbs: 4.1g
- Protein: 4.4g

53. Raspberry Dump Cake

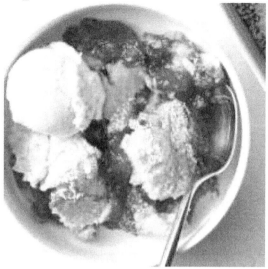

Preparation time: 10 minutes
Cooking time: 30 minutes
Servings: 10
Ingredients:

- ½ cup raspberries
- 1 ½ cup coconut flour
- ⅓ cup almond milk
- ¼ cup Erythritol
- 1 egg; whisked - 1 tbsp. butter; melted
- 1 tsp. baking powder
- ½ tsp. vanilla extract
- 1 tsp. lemon juice

Directions:

1. Combine together all the dry ingredients. Then add egg, almond milk, and butter Add vanilla extract and lemon juice. Stir the mixture well. You have to get a liquid batter.
2. Place the layer of the raspberries in the silicone mold. Pour batter over the raspberries. Place the mold on the rack and insert it into the Ninja Foodi basket.
3. Close the air fryer lid and set Bake mode. Cook the cake for 30 minutes at 350°F. When the cake is cooked; chill it well. Turn upside down and transfer on the serving plate.

Nutrition:

- Calories: 107 Fat: 4.5g Carbs: 15.1g Protein: 4.3g

54. Pumpkin Pie

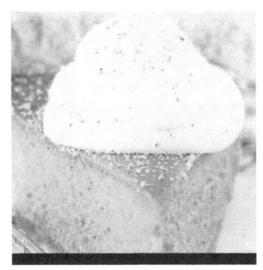

Preparation time: 10 minutes
Cooking time: 25 minutes
Servings: 6
Ingredients:

- 1 cup coconut flour
- ¼ cup heavy cream
- 1 egg; whisked
- 1 tbsp. butter
- 2 tbsps. liquid stevia
- 1 tbsp. pumpkin puree
- 1 tsp. apple cider vinegar
- 1 tsp. Pumpkin spices
- ½ tsp. baking powder

Directions:

1. Melt the butter and combine it together with the heavy cream, apple cider vinegar, liquid stevia, egg, and baking powder
2. Add pumpkin puree and coconut flour. Now, add pumpkin spices and stir the batter until smooth.
3. Pour the batter in Ninja Foodi basket and lower the air fryer lid
4. Set the "Bake" mode 360°F. Cook the pie for 25 minutes. When the time is over; let the pie chill till room temperature.

Nutrition:

- Calories: 127 Fat: 6.6g Carbs: 14.2g Protein: 3.8g

55. Avocado Mousse

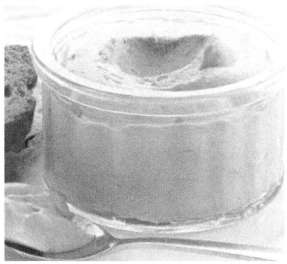

Preparation time: 2 minutes
Cooking time: 10 minutes
Servings: 7
Ingredients:

- 2 avocados, peeled, cored
- 3 tbsps. Erythritol
- ⅓ cup heavy cream
- 1 tsp. butter
- 1 tsp. vanilla extract
- 1 tsp. of cocoa powder

Directions:

1. Preheat Ninja Foodi at "Sauté" mode for 5 minutes. Meanwhile, mash the avocado until smooth and mix it up with Erythritol
2. Place the butter in the pot and melt. Add mashed avocado mixture and stir well.
3. Add cocoa powder and stir until homogenous. Sauté the mixture for 3 minutes
4. Meanwhile, whisk the heavy cream at high speed for 2 minutes. Transfer the cooked avocado mash to the bowl and chill in ice water.
5. When the avocado mash reaches room temperature; add whisked heavy cream and vanilla extract. Stir gently to get white chocolate swirls
6. Transfer the mousse into small cups and chill for 4 hours in the fridge.

Nutrition:

- Calories: 144 Fat: 13.9g
- Carbs: 10.5g Protein: 1.3g

56. Almond Bites

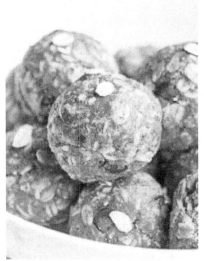

Preparation time: 10 minutes
Cooking time: 14 minutes
Servings: 5
Ingredients:

- 1 cup almond flour
- ¼ cup almond milk
- 1 egg; whisked
- 2 tbsps. butter
- 1 tbsp. coconut flakes
- ½ tsp. baking powder
- ½ tsp. apple cider vinegar
- ½ tsp. vanilla extract

Directions:

1. Mix up together the whisked egg, almond milk, apple cider vinegar, baking powder, vanilla extract, and butter.
2. Stir the mixture and add almond flour and coconut flakes. Knead the dough.
3. If the dough is sticky; add more almond flour. Make the medium balls from the dough and place them on the rack of Ninja Foodi.
4. Press them gently with the hand palm. Lower the air fryer lid and cook the dessert for 12 minutes at 360°F.
5. Check if the dessert is cooked; and cook for 2 minutes more for a crunchy crust.

Nutrition:

- Calories: 118 Fat: 11.5g Carbs: 2.4g Protein: 2.7g

57. Mint Cake

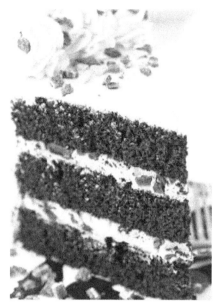

Preparation time: 10 minutes
Cooking time: 1 hour
Servings: 6
Ingredients:

- ¼ cup Erythritol
- 2 eggs; whisked
- ¼ cup heavy cream
- 1 cup coconut flour
- 1 tbsp. butter
- ½ tsp. lemon zest; grated
- 1 tsp. dried mint
- 1 tsp. baking powder

Directions:

1. In the mixing bowl mix up together all the ingredients. Use the cooking machine to make the soft batter from the mixture.
2. Pour the batter into the Ninja Foodie basket and flatten it well. Close the pressure cooker lid and set Pressure mode. Seal the lid.
3. Cook the cake on Low pressure for 55 minutes. Then lower the air fryer lid and set Air Crisp mode.
4. Cook the cake for 7 minutes more at 400°F. Chill the cake well and serve!

Nutrition:

- Calories: 136 Fat: 7.2g Carbs: 22g Protein: 4.7g

58. Brownie Batter

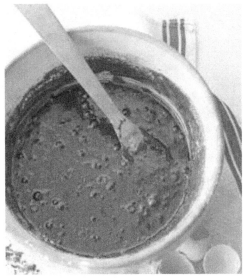

Preparation time: 5 minutes
Cooking time: 4 minutes
Servings: 5
Ingredients:

- 1 oz. dark chocolate - ¼ cup heavy cream
- ⅓ cup almond flour
- 1 tbsp. Erythritol
- 3 tbsps. cocoa powder
- 3 tbsps. butter
- ½ tsp. vanilla extract

Directions:

1. Place the almond flour in the springform pan and flatten to make the layer. Then place the springform pan in the pot and lower the air fryer lid
2. Cook the almond flour for 3 minutes at 400°F or until the almond flour gets a golden color.
3. Meanwhile, combine together cocoa powder and heavy cream; whisk the heavy cream until smooth
4. Add vanilla extract and Erythritol. Remove the almond flour from Ninja Foodi and chill well.
5. Toss butter and dark chocolate in the pot and preheat for 1 minute on Sauté mode When the butter is soft; add it to the heavy cream mixture. Then add chocolate and almond flour. Stir the mass until homogenous and serve!

Nutrition:

- Calories: 159 Fat: 14.9g Carbs: 9g Protein: 2.5g

59. Peanut Butter Cookies

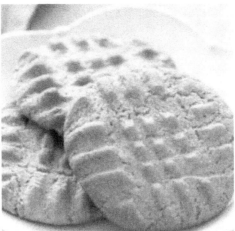

Preparation time: 10 minutes
Cooking time: 11 minutes
Servings: 7
Ingredients:

- 6 oz. cashew butter
- 1 egg; whisked
- 1 tbsp. Truvia

Directions:

1. Mix up together all the ingredients and make the small balls. Place the balls in the basket of Ninja Foodi and close the lid
2. Set the Bake mode and cook the cookies at 330°F for 11 minutes. Increase the time of cooking if you like crunchy cookies

Nutrition:

- Calories: 152
- Fat: 12.6g
- Carbs: 7.4g
- Protein: 5.1g

60. Vanilla Custard

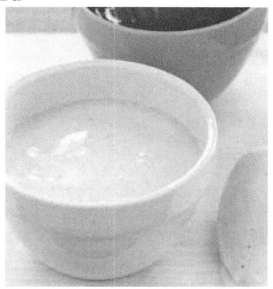

Preparation time: 5 minutes
Cooking time: 15 minutes
Servings: 4
Ingredients:

- 1 cup almond milk
- 3 egg yolks
- 2 tbsps. Truvia
- 1 tsp. vanilla extract

Directions:

1. Whisk together egg yolk and Truvia. Add vanilla extract and almond milk
2. Preheat Ninja Foodi at Sauté mode at 365°F for 5 minutes
3. Then pour the almond milk mixture and Sauté it for 10 minutes.
4. Stir the liquid all the time. When the liquid start to be thick; transfer it into the serving jars and leave it for 1 hour in the fridge

Nutrition:

- Calories: 181
- Fat: 17.7g
- Carbs: 6.2g
- Protein: 3.4g

61. Crunchy Chicken Skin

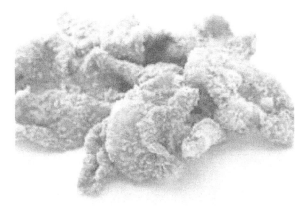

Preparation time: 10 minutes
Cooking time: 10 minutes
Servings: 7
Ingredients:

- 1 tsp. red chili flakes
- 1 tsp. ground black pepper
- 1 tsp. salt
- 9 oz. chicken's skin
- 2 tbsps. butter
- 1 tsp. organic essential olive oil
- 1 tsp. paprika

Directions:

1. Combine black pepper, salt with chili flakes, and paprika. Stir.
2. Combine the mixture with chicken skin and let it rest for 5 minutes.
3. Set the pressure cooker to sauté mode and add butter.
4. Immediately the butter melts, add the chicken skin and sauté it for 10 minutes while stirring frequently. When the chicken skin gets crunchy, take it off from the pressure cooker and place it on a paper towel to drain excess oils.
5. Serve warm.

Nutrition:

- Calories: 134
- Carbs: 0.98g
- Fat: 11.5g
- Protein: 7g

62. Meatloaf

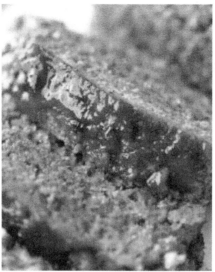

Preparation time: 10 minutes
Cooking time: 40 minutes
Servings: 9
Ingredients:

- 2 cups, ground beef
- 1 cup, ground chicken
- 2 eggs - 1 tbsps. salt
- 1 tsp. ground black pepper
- ½ tsp. paprika - 1 tbsps. butter
- 1 tsp. cilantro - 1 tbsps. basil
- ¼ cup, fresh dill
- Breadcrumbs

Directions:

1. Combine chicken with ground beef in a mixing bowl.
2. Add egg, salt, ground black pepper, paprika, butter, cilantro, and basil.
3. Chop the dill and add it to the ground meat mixture and stir using your hand.
4. Place the meat mixture on an aluminum foil and add breadcrumbs before wrapping it. Place it in a pressure cooker and close its lid. Cook the dish in sauté mode and cook for 40 minutes.
5. When the cooking time ends, remove your meatloaf from the cooker and allow it to cool. Unwrap the foil, slice it, and serve.

Nutrition:

- Calories: 173 Fat: 11.5g Carbs: 0.81g Protein: 16g

CHAPTER 13:

Salads & Soups

63. Butternut Squash Soup

Preparation time: 10 minutes
Cooking time: 8 hours
Servings: 9
Ingredients:

- 2 lb. butternut squash
- 4 tsps. minced garlic
- ½ cup onion, chopped
- 1 tsp. salt
- ¼ tsp. ground nutmeg
- 1 tsp. ground black pepper
- 8 cups chicken stock
- 1 tbsp. fresh parsley

Directions:

1. Peel the butternut squash and cut it into chunks.
2. Toss the butternut squash in the slow cooker.
3. Add chopped onion, minced garlic, and chicken stock.
4. Close the slow cooker lid and cook the soup for 8 hours on LOW.
5. Meanwhile, combine the ground black pepper, ground nutmeg, and salt together.
6. Chop the fresh parsley.
7. When the time is done, remove the soup from the slow cooker and blend it with a blender until you get a creamy soup.
8. Sprinkle the soup with the spice mixture and add chopped parsley. Serve the soup warm. Enjoy!

Nutrition:

- Calories: 129 Fat: 2.7g
- Fiber: 2g Carbs: 20.85g Protein: 7g

INTERMITTENT FASTING FOR WOMEN OVER 50

64. Eggplant Bacon Wraps

Preparation time: 17 minutes
Cooking time: 5 hours
Servings: 6
Ingredients:

- 10 oz. eggplant, sliced into rounds
- 5 oz. halloumi cheese
- 1 tsp. minced garlic
- 3 oz. bacon, chopped
- ½ tsp. ground black pepper
- 1 tsp. salt
- 1 tsp. paprika
- 1 tomato

Directions:

1. Rub the eggplant slices with the ground black pepper, salt, and paprika.
2. Slice halloumi cheese and tomato.
3. Combine the chopped bacon and minced garlic together.
4. Place the sliced eggplants in the slow cooker. Cook the eggplant on HIGH for 1 hour.
5. Chill the eggplant. Place the sliced tomato and cheese on the eggplant slices.
6. Add the chopped bacon mixture and roll up tightly.
7. Secure the eggplants with the toothpicks and return the eggplant wraps back into the slow cooker. Cook the dish on HIGH for 4 hours more.
8. When the dish is done, serve it immediately. Enjoy!

Nutrition:

- Calories: 131
- Fat: 9.4g
- Fiber: 2g
- Carbs: 7.25g
- Protein: 6g

65. Mexican Warm Salad

Preparation time: 26 minutes
Cooking time: 10 hours
Servings: 10
Ingredients:

- 1 cup black beans
- 1 cup sweet corn, frozen
- 3 tomatoes
- 1 chili pepper
- 7 oz. chicken fillet
- 5 oz. Cheddar cheese
- 4 tbsps. mayonnaise
- 1 tsp. minced garlic
- 1 cup lettuce
- 5 cups chicken stock
- 1 cucumber

Directions:

1. Put the chicken fillet, sweet corn, black beans, and chicken stock in the slow cooker.
2. Close the slow cooker lid and cook the mixture on LOW for 10 hours.
3. When the time is done remove the mixture from the slow cooker.
4. Shred the chicken fillet with 2 forks. Chill the mixture until room temperature.
5. Chop the lettuce roughly. Chop the cucumber and tomatoes.
6. Place the lettuce, cucumber, and tomatoes on a large serving plate.
7. After this, shred Cheddar cheese and chop the chili pepper.
8. Add the chili pepper to the serving plate too.
9. After this, add the chicken mixture to the top of the salad.
10. Sprinkle the salad with mayonnaise, minced garlic, and shredded cheese. Enjoy the salad immediately.

Nutrition:

- Calories: 182
- Fat: 7.8g
- Fiber: 2g
- Carbs: 19.6g
- Protein: 9g

66.   Hot Chorizo Salad

Preparation time: 20 minutes
Cooking time: 4 hours 30 minutes
Servings: 6
Ingredients:

- 8 oz. chorizo
- 1 tsp. olive oil
- 1 tsp. cayenne pepper
- 1 tsp. chili flakes
- 1 tsp. ground black pepper
- 1 tsp. onion powder
- 2 garlic cloves
- 3 tomatoes
- 1 cup lettuce
- 1 cup fresh dill
- 1 tsp. oregano
- 3 tbsps. crushed cashews

Directions:

1. Chop the chorizo sausages roughly and place them in the slow cooker.
2. Cook the sausages for 4 hours on HIGH.
3. Meanwhile, combine the cayenne pepper, chili flakes, ground black pepper, and onion powder together in a shallow bowl.
4. Chop the tomatoes roughly and add them to the slow cooker after 4 hours. Cook the mixture for 30 minutes more on HIGH.
5. Chop the fresh dill and combine it with oregano.
6. When the chorizo sausage mixture is cooked, place it in a serving bowl. Tear the lettuce and add it to the bowl too.
7. After this, peel the garlic cloves and slice them.
8. Add the sliced garlic cloves to the salad bowl too.
9. Then sprinkle the salad with the spice mixture, olive oil, fresh dill mixture, and crush cashew. Mix the salad carefully. Enjoy!

Nutrition:

- Calories: 249
- Fat: 19.8g
- Fiber: 2g
- Carbs: 7.69g
- Protein: 11g

67. Ham Soup

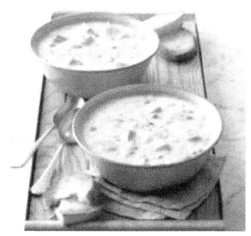

Preparation time: 5 minutes
Cooking time: 4 hours
Servings: 6
Ingredients:

- 2 lbs. pasture-raised smoked ham hock
- 2 cups cauliflower florets
- 2 bay leaves
- ¼ tsp. nutmeg
- cups bone broth

Directions:

1. Place cauliflower florets in a 6-quarts slow cooker, add remaining ingredients, and pour in water until all the ingredients are just submerged.
2. Plug in the slow cooker then shut with lid and cook for 4 hours at a high heat setting or until cauliflower florets are very tender.
3. Transfer ham to a bowl, shred with two forms and discard bone and fat pieces.
4. Puree cauliflower in the slow cooker with a stick blender for 1 to 2 minutes or until smooth, return shredded ham and stir until well combined.
5. Taste soup to adjust seasoning and serve.

Nutrition:

- Carbs: 3g
- Calories: 349
- Total Fat: 23g
- Saturated Fat: 10g
- Protein: 34g
- Fiber: 2g Sugar: 2g

CHAPTER 14:

Meat recipes

68. Stuffed Beef Loin in Sticky Sauce

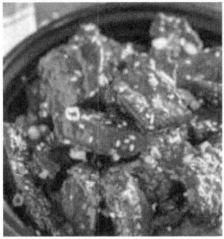

Preparation time: 15 minutes
Cooking time: 6 minutes
Servings: 4
Ingredients:

- 1 tbsp. Erythritol
- 1 tbsp. lemon juice
- 4 tbsps. water
- 1 tbsp. butter
- ½ tsp. tomato sauce
- ¼ tsp. dried rosemary
- 9 oz. beef loin
- 3 oz. celery root, grated
- 3 oz. bacon, sliced
- 1 tbsp. walnuts, chopped
- ¾ tsp. garlic, diced
- 2 tsps. butter
- 1 tbsp. olive oil

- 1 tsp. salt
- ½ cup of water

Directions:

1. Cut the beef loin into the layer and spread it with the dried rosemary, butter, and salt.
2. Then place over the beef loin: grated celery root, sliced bacon, walnuts, and diced garlic.
3. Roll the beef loin and brush it with olive oil.
4. Secure the meat with the help of the toothpicks.
5. Place it in the tray and add a ½ cup of water.
6. Cook the meat in the preheated to 365F oven for 40 minutes.
7. Meanwhile, make the sticky sauce: mix up together Erythritol, lemon juice, 4 tablespoons of water, and butter.
8. Preheat the mixture until it starts to boil.
9. Then add tomato sauce and whisk it well.
10. Bring the sauce to a boil and remove it from the heat.
11. When the beef loin is cooked, remove it from the oven and brush it with the cooked sticky sauce very generously.
12. Slice the beef roll and sprinkle with the remaining sauce.

Nutrition:

- Calories: 215
- Protein: 8.7g
- Carbs: 18.5g
- Fat: 11.5g
- Fiber: 2.3g

69. Pork Chops

Preparation time: 5 minutes
Cooking time: 6 hours
Servings: 8
Ingredients:

- 2 lbs. pasture-raised pork chops
- 1 tsp. salt
- 1 tbsp. dried thyme
- 1 tbsp. dried rosemary
- 1 tbsp. ground cumin
- 1 tbsp. dried curry powder
- 1 tbsp. chopped fresh chives
- 1 tbsp. fennel seeds
- 1 tbsp. avocado oil

Directions:

1. Place 2 tbsps. oil in a small bowl, add remaining ingredients except for pork and stir until well mixed.
2. Rub this mixture on all sides of pork chops until evenly coated.
3. Grease a 6-quart slow cooker with remaining oil, add seasoned pork chops, and shut with lid.
4. Plug in the slow cooker and cook pork for 6 hours at a low heat setting or 4 hours at a high heat setting.
5. Serve straight away.

Nutrition:

- Carbs: 1g
- Calories: 235
- Total Fat: 15g
- Saturated Fat: 3g
- Protein: 24g
- Fiber: 0g
- Sugar: 0g

70. Spicy Pork & Spinach Stew

Preparation time: 5 minutes
Cooking time: 4 hours and 20 minutes
Servings: 5
Ingredients:

- 1 lb. pasture-raised pork butt, fat trimmed and cut into 2-inch pieces
- 4 cups chopped baby spinach
- 4 oz. Rotel tomatoes
- 1 large white onion, peeled and quartered
- cloves of garlic, peeled
- 1 tsp. dried thyme
- 2 tsps. Cajun seasoning blend
- 2 tbsps. avocado oil
- ¾ cup heavy whipping cream

Directions:

1. Place tomatoes, onion, and garlic in a food processor and pulse for 1 to 2 minutes or until blended.
2. Pour this mixture into a 6-quart slow cooker, add Cajun seasoning mix, thyme, avocado oil, and pork pieces, and stir well until evenly coated.
3. Plug in the slow cooker, then shut with lid and cook for 5 hours at low heat setting or 2 hours at high heat setting.
4. When done, stir in cream until combined, add spinach and continue cooking at low heat setting for 20 minutes or more until spinach wilts.
5. Serve straight away.

Nutrition:

- Calories: 604
- Total Fat: 38.3g
- Saturated Fat: 9g
- Protein: 56g
- Carbs: 9g
- Fiber: 5g
- Sugar: 4g

71. Lamb Barbacoa

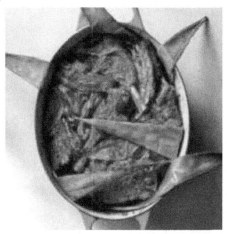

Preparation time: 5 minutes
Cooking time: 8 hours
Servings: 12
Ingredients:

- 2 lbs. pasture-raised pork shoulder, fat trimmed
- 2 tbsps. salt
- 1 tsp. chipotle powder
- 2 tbsps. smoked paprika
- 1 tbsp. ground cumin
- 1 tbsp. dried oregano
- ¼ cup dried mustard
- 1 cup water

Directions:

1. Stir together salt, chipotle powder, paprika, cumin, oregano, and mustard and rub this mixture generously all over the pork.
2. Place seasoned pork into a 6-quart slow cooker, plug it in, then shut with lid and cook for 6 hours at high heat setting.
3. When done, shred pork with two forks and stir well until coated well.
4. Serve straight away.

Nutrition:

- Calories: 477
- Total Fat: 35.8g
- Saturated Fat: 14.8g
- Protein: 37.5g
- Carbs: 1.2g Fiber: 0.5g
- Sugar: 5g

72. Pork Chile Verde

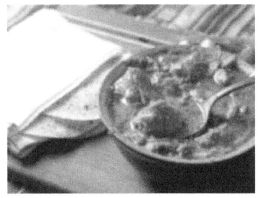

Preparation time: 5 minutes
Cooking time: 7 hours and 5 minutes
Servings: 6
Ingredients:

- 2 lbs. pasture-raised pork shoulder, cut into 6 pieces
- 1 tsp. sea salt
- ½ tsp. ground black pepper
- 1 ½ tbsp. avocado oil
- 1 ½ cup salsa Verde
- 1 cup chicken broth

Directions:

1. Season pork with salt and black pepper.
2. Place a large skillet pans over medium heat, add oil, and when hot, add seasoned pork pieces.
3. Cook pork for 3 to 4 minutes per side or until browned and then transfer to a 6-quart slow cooker.
4. Whisk together salsa and chicken broth and pour over pork pieces.
5. Plug in the slow cooker then shut with lid and cook for 6 to 7 hours at low heat setting or until pork is very tender.
6. When done, shred pork with two forks and stir until combined.

Nutrition:

- Calories: 342
- Total Fat: 22g
- Saturated Fat: 12g
- Protein: 32g
- Carbs: 6g
- Fiber: 2g
- Sugar: 4g

73. Minced Pork Zucchini Lasagna

Preparation time: 20 minutes
Cooking time: 8 hours
Servings: 4
Ingredients:

- 2 medium zucchinis
- 1 diced small onion
- 1 minced clove of garlic
- 2 cups of minced lean ground pork
- 2 cans of Italian diced tomatoes
- 2 tbsps. of olive oil
- 2 cups of shredded Mozzarella cheese
- 1 large egg
- 2 tbsps. of butter

Directions:

1. Slice the zucchini lengthwise into 6 slices.
2. Heat the olive oil in a saucepan and sauté the garlic and onions for 5 minutes.
3. Add the minced meat and cook for a further 5 minutes.
4. Add the tomatoes and cook for a further 5 minutes.
5. Add the seasoning and mix thoroughly.
6. In a small bowl, combine the egg and cheese and whisk together.
7. Use the butter to grease the crockpot and then begin to layer the lasagna.
8. First, layer with the zucchini slices, add the meat mixture and then top with the cheese.
9. Repeat and finish with the cheese.
10. Cover and cook for 8 hours on low.

Nutrition:

- Carbs: 10g
- Protein: 23g
- Fat: 30g
- Calories: 398

74. Beef Dijon

Preparation time: 15 minutes
Cooking time: 5 hours
Servings: 4
Ingredients:

- 6 oz. small round steaks
- 2 tbsps. steak seasoning (to taste)
- 2 tbsps. avocado oil
- 2 tbsps. peanut oil
- 2 tbsps. balsamic vinegar/dry sherry
- 2 large chopped green onions/small chopped onions for the garnish (extra)
- ¼ cup whipping cream
- 1 cup fresh crimini mushrooms, sliced
- 1 tbsp. Dijon mustard

Directions:

1. Warm up the oils using the high heat setting on the stovetop. Flavor each of the steaks with pepper and arrange to a skillet.
2. Cook two to three minutes per side until done.
3. Place into the slow cooker. Pour in the skillet drippings, half of the mushrooms, and the onions.
4. Cook on the low setting for four hours.
5. When the cooking time is done, scoop out the onions, mushrooms, and steaks to a serving platter.
6. In a separate dish—whisk together the mustard, balsamic vinegar, whipping cream, and the steak drippings from the slow cooker.
7. Empty the gravy into a gravy server and pour over the steaks.
8. Enjoy with some brown rice, riced cauliflower, or potatoes.

Nutrition:

- Calories: 535
- Carbs: 5.0g
- Fat: 40g
- Protein: 39g

75. Cabbage & Corned Beef

Preparation time: 10 minutes
Cooking time: 8 hours
Servings: 10
Ingredients:

- 1 lb. corned beef
- 1 large head cabbage
- 1 cup water
- 1 celery bunch
- 1 small onion
- 4 carrots
- ½ tsp. ground mustard
- ½ tsp. ground coriander
- ½ tsp. ground marjoram
- ½ tsp. black pepper
- ½ tsp. salt
- ½ tsp. ground thyme
- ½ tsp. allspice

Directions:

1. Dice the carrots, onions, and celery and toss them into the cooker. Pour in the water.
2. Combine the spices, rub the beef, and arrange in the cooker. Secure the lid and cook on low for seven hours.
3. Remove the top layer of cabbage. Wash and cut it into quarters until ready to cook. When the beef is done, add the cabbage, and cook for one hour on the low setting.
4. Serve and enjoy.

Nutrition:

- Calories: 583
- Carbs: 13g
- Fat: 40g
- Protein: 42g

CHAPTER 15:

Fish Recipes

76. Fried Codfish with Almonds

Preparation time: 8 minutes
Cooking time: 18 minutes
Servings: 3
Ingredients:

- 16 oz. codfish fillet
- 3 oz. chopped almonds
- ½ tsp. chili pepper
- 1 egg
- 1 tbsp. ghee butter
- 1 tsp. psyllium
- 3 oz. cream
- 1 tbsp. chopped fresh dill
- 1 tsp. minced garlic
- ½ tsp. onion powder
- Salt and pepper to taste

Directions:

1. In a small mixing bowl, combine the psyllium, onion powder, chili, and almonds
2. Beat the egg in another bowl, mix well
3. Warm the butter in a skillet at medium heat.
4. Cut the fillet into 3 slices
5. Dip into the egg mixture, then into almonds and spices
6. Fry in the skillet for about 7 minutes on each side
7. Meanwhile, in another bowl combine the cream, garlic, dill, and salt, stir well
8. Serve the fish with this sauce.

Nutrition:

- Carbs: 4,9g
- Fat: 63g
- Protein: 33,6g
- Calories: 709

77. Salmon Balls
Preparation time: 5 minutes
Cooking time: 13 minutes
Servings: 2
Ingredients:
- 1 can salmon
- 2 tbsps. intermittent mayo
- 1 avocado
- 1 egg
- 1 garlic clove
- ½ cup heavy cream
- 3 tbsps. coconut oil
- ½ tsp. ginger powder
- ½ tsp. paprika
- ½ tsp. dried cilantro
- 2 tbsps. lemon juice
- 2 tbsps. water
- Salt and ground black pepper to taste

Directions:
1. Drain the salmon, chop it
2. Mince the garlic clove, peel the avocado
3. In a bowl, combine the fish, mayo, egg, and garlic, season with salt, paprika, and ginger, mix well
4. Make 4 balls of it
5. Warm the oil in a skillet at medium heat
6. Put the balls and fry for 4-6 minutes on each side
7. Meanwhile, put the heavy cream, avocado, cilantro, lemon juice, and 1 tablespoon of oil in a blender. Pulse well
8. Serve the balls with the sauce.

Nutrition:
- Carbs: 3,9g
- Fat: 50g
- Protein: 20,1g
- Calories: 555

78. Codfish Sticks

Preparation time: 8 minutes
Cooking time: 15 minutes
Servings: 2
Ingredients:

- 9 oz. codfish fillet
- 2 eggs
- 2 tbsps. ghee butter
- 2 tbsps. coconut flour
- ½ tsp. paprika
- Salt and pepper to taste

Directions:

1. Slice the fish into sticks
2. In a bowl, put and mix the eggs, flour, paprika, pepper, and salt
3. Warm the butter in a skillet at medium heat.
4. Dip each fish slice into the spice mixture
5. Fry in the skillet over low heat for 4-5 minutes per side.

Nutrition:

- Carbs: 1,5g
- Fat: 31g
- Protein: 22,5g
- Calories: 329

79. Shrimp Risotto

Preparation time: 10 minutes

Cooking time: 15 minutes

Servings: 4

Ingredients:

- 14 oz. shrimps, peeled and deveined
- 12 oz. cauli rice
- 4 button mushrooms
- ½ lemon
- 4 stalks green onion
- 3 tbsps. ghee butter
- 2 tbsps. coconut oil
- Salt and black pepper to taste

Directions:

1. Preheat the oven to 400°F
2. Put a layer of cauli rice on a sheet pan, season with salt and spices; sprinkle the coconut oil over it
3. Bake in the oven for 10-12 minutes
4. Cut the green onion, slice up the mushrooms and remove the rind from the lemon
5. Heat the ghee butter in a skillet over medium heat. Add the shrimps; season it and sauté for 5-6 minutes
6. Top the cauli rice with the shrimps, sprinkle the green onion over it.

Nutrition:

- Carbs: 9,2g
- Fat: 26,2g
- Protein: 25g
- Calories: 363

80. Lemony Trout

Preparation time: 10 minutes

Cooking time: 20 minutes

Servings: 2

Ingredients:

- 5 tbsp. ghee butter
- 5 oz. trout fillets
- 2 garlic cloves
- 1 tsp. rosemary
- 1 lemon
- 2 tbsps. capers
- Salt and pepper to taste

Directions:

1. Preheat the oven to 400°F
2. Peel the lemon, mince the garlic cloves and chop the capers
3. Season the trout fillets with salt, rosemary, and pepper
4. Grease a baking dish with the oil and place the fish onto it
5. Warm the butter in a skillet over medium heat
6. Add the garlic and cook for 4-5 minutes until golden
7. Remove from the heat, add the lemon zest and 2 tablespoons of lemon juice, stir well
8. Pour the lemon-butter sauce over the fish and top with the capers
9. Bake for 14-15 minutes. Serve hot.

Nutrition:

- Carbs: 3,1g
- Fat: 25g
- Protein: 15,8g
- Calories: 302

81. Quick Fish Bowl

Preparation time: 11 minutes
Cooking time: 15 minutes
Servings: 2
Ingredients:

- 2 tilapia fillets
- 1 tbsp. olive oil
- 1 avocado
- 1 tbsp. ghee butter
- 1 tbsp. cumin powder
- 1 tbsp. paprika
- 2 cups coleslaw cabbage, chopped
- 1 tbsp. salsa sauce
- Himalayan rock salt, to taste
- Black pepper to taste

Directions:

1. Preheat the oven to 425°F. Line a baking sheet with the foil
2. Mash the avocado
3. Brush the tilapia fillets using olive oil, season with salt and spices
4. Place the fish onto the baking sheet, greased with the ghee butter
5. Bake for 15 minutes, then remove the fish from the heat and let it cool for 5 minutes
6. In a bowl, combine the coleslaw cabbage and the salsa sauce, toss gently
7. Add the mashed avocado, season with salt and pepper
8. Slice the fish and add to the bowl
9. Bake for 14-15 minutes. Serve hot.

Nutrition:

- Carbs: 5,2g
- Fat: 24,5g
- Protein: 16,1g
- Calories: 321

82. Omelet Wrap with Avocado and Salmon

Preparation time: 10 minutes
Cooking time: 6 minutes
Servings: 2
Ingredients:

- 1 avocado, sliced
- 2 tbsps. chopped chives
- 2 oz. smoked salmon, sliced
- 1 spring onion, sliced
- 4 eggs, beaten
- 3 tbsps. cream cheese
- 2 tbsps. butter
- Salt and black pepper to taste

Directions:

1. In a small bowl, combine the chives and cream cheese; set aside. Season the eggs with salt and pepper. Melt butter in a pan and add the eggs; cook for 3 minutes.
2. Flip the omelet over and cook for another 2 minutes until golden.
3. Remove to a plate and spread the chive mixture over. Top with salmon, avocado, and onion slices. Wrap and serve.

Nutrition:

- Calories: 514
- Carbs: 5.8g
- Fat: 47g
- Protein: 37g

CHAPTER 16:

Superfoods for Women over 50

83. Roasted Brussels Sprouts with Pecans and Gorgonzola

Preparation time: 10 minutes
Cooking time: 35 minutes
Servings: 4
Ingredients:

- 1 lb. Brussels Sprouts, fresh
- ¼ cup Pecans, chopped
- 1 tbsp. Olive oil (Extra olive oil to oil the baking tray)
- Pepper and salt for tasting
- ¼ cup Gorgonzola cheese (If you prefer not to use the Gorgonzola cheese, you can toss the Brussels sprouts when hot, with 2 tbsps. of butter instead.)

Directions:

1. Warm the oven to 350°F or 175°C.
2. Rub a large pan or any vessel you wish to use with a little bit of olive oil. You can use a paper towel or a pastry brush.
3. Cut off the ends of the Brussels sprouts if you need to and then cut them in a lengthwise direction into halves. (Fear not if a few of the leaves come off of them, some may become deliciously crunchy during cooking)
4. Chop up all of the pecans using a knife and then measure them for the amount.
5. Put your Brussels sprouts as well as the sliced pecans inside a bowl, and cover them all with some olive oil, pepper, and salt (be generous).
6. Arrange all of your pecans and Brussels sprouts onto your roasting pan in a single layer
7. Roast this for 30 to 35 minutes, or when they become tender and can be pierced with a fork easily. Stir during cooking if you wish to get a more even browning.
8. Once cooked, toss them with the Gorgonzola Cheese (or butter) before you serve them. Serve them hot.

Nutrition:

- Calories: 149
- Fat: 11g Protein: 5g

84. Stuffed Beef Loin in Sticky Sauce

Preparation time: 15 minutes
Cooking time: 6 minutes
Servings: 4
Ingredients:

- 1 tbsp. Erythritol
- 1 tbsp. lemon juice
- ½ tsp. tomato sauce
- ¼ tsp. dried rosemary
- 9 oz. beef loin
- 3 oz. celery root, grated
- 3 oz. bacon, sliced
- 1 tbsp. walnuts, chopped
- ¾ tsp. garlic, diced
- 2 tsps. butter
- 1 tbsp. olive oil
- 1 tsp. salt
- ½ cup of water

Directions:

1. Cut the beef loin into the layer and spread it with the dried rosemary, butter, and salt. Then place over the beef loin: grated celery root, sliced bacon, walnuts, and diced garlic.
2. Roll the beef loin and brush it with olive oil. Secure the meat with the help of the toothpicks. Place it in the tray and add a ½ cup of water.
3. Cook the meat in the preheated to 365°F oven for 40 minutes.
4. Meanwhile, make the sticky sauce:
5. Mix up together Erythritol, lemon juice, 4 tablespoons of water, and butter.
6. Preheat the mixture until it starts to boil. Then add tomato sauce and whisk it well.
7. Bring the sauce to a boil and remove it from the heat.
8. When the beef loin is cooked, remove it from the oven and brush it with the cooked sticky sauce very generously.
9. Slice the beef roll and sprinkle with the remaining sauce.

Nutrition:

- Calories: 321
- Protein: 18.35g
- Fat: 26.68g

85. Eggplant Fries

Preparation time: 10 minutes
Cooking time: 15 minutes
Servings: 8
Ingredients:

- 2 eggs
- 2 cups almond flour
- 2 tbsps. coconut oil, spray
- 2 eggplant, peeled and cut thinly
- Salt and pepper

Directions:

1. Preheat your oven to 400°F
2. Take a bowl and mix with salt and black pepper in it
3. Take another bowl and beat eggs until frothy
4. Dip the eggplant pieces into eggs
5. Then coat them with a flour mixture
6. Add another layer of flour and egg
7. Then, take a baking sheet and grease with coconut oil on top
8. Bake for about 15 minutes
9. Serve and enjoy.

Nutrition:

- Calories: 212
- Fat: 15.8g
- Protein: 8.6g

86. Parmesan Crisps

Preparation time: 5 minutes
Cooking time: 25 minutes
Servings: 8
Ingredients:

- 1 tsp. butter
- 8 oz. parmesan cheese, full fat, and shredded

Directions:

1. Preheat your oven to 400°F
2. Put parchment paper on a baking sheet and grease with butter
3. Spoon parmesan into 8 mounds, spreading them apart evenly
4. Flatten them
5. Bake for 5 minutes until browned
6. Let them cool
7. Serve and enjoy.

Nutrition:

- Calories: 133
- Fat: 11g
- Protein: 11g

87. Roasted Broccoli

Preparation time: 5 minutes
Cooking time: 20 minutes
Servings: 4
Ingredients:

- 4 cups broccoli florets
- 1 tbsp. olive oil
- Salt and pepper to taste

Directions:

1. Preheat your oven to 400°F
2. Add broccoli in a zip bag alongside oil and shake until coated
3. Add seasoning and shake again
4. Spread broccoli out on the baking sheet, bake for 20 minutes
5. Let it cool and serve.

Nutrition:

- Calories: 62
- Fat: 4g
- Protein: 4g

88. Almond Flour Muffins

Preparation time: 15 minutes
Cooking time: 30 minutes
Servings: 8
Ingredients:

- ⅓ cup of pumpkin puree
- 3 eggs
- 2 tbsps. agave nectar
- 2 tbsps. coconut oil
- 1 tsp. vanilla extract
- 1 tsp. white vinegar
- 1 cup chopped fruits
- 1 tsp. baking soda
- ½ tsp. salt
- 1 cup almond flour

Directions:

1. Preheat the oven to 350°F.
2. Line the muffin tin with paper liners
3. In the first mixing bowl, whisk the almond flour, salt, and baking soda.
4. In the second mixing bowl, whisk the pumpkin puree, eggs, coconut oil, agave nectar, vanilla extract, and vinegar.
5. Now add this puree mix of the second bowl to the first bowl and blend everything well.
6. Add the chopped fruits to the blend.
7. Pour the mixture into the muffin cups in your pan.
8. Bake for 15-20 minutes. Ensure that the contents have set in the center, and a golden brown lining has started to appear at the edges.
9. Transfer the muffins to a cooling rack and let them cool completely.

Nutrition:

- Calories: 75
- Fat: 6g
- Protein: 0g

89. Squash Bites

Preparation time: 10 minutes
Cooking time: 40 minutes
Servings: 4
Ingredients:

- 10 oz. of turkey meat, cooked, sliced
- 2 lbs. butternut squash, cubed
- 1 tsp. chili powder
- 1 tsp. garlic powder
- 1 tsp. sweet paprika
- Black pepper to taste

Directions:

1. In a bowl, mix butternut squash cubes with chili powder, black pepper, garlic powder, and paprika and toss to coat.
2. Wrap squash pieces in turkey slices, place them all on a lined baking sheet, place in the oven at 350°F, bake for 20 minutes, flip and bake for 20 minutes more.
3. Arrange squash bites on a platter and serve. Enjoy

Nutrition:

- Calories: 223
- Fat: 3.8g
- Protein: 23g

90. Zucchini Chips

Preparation time: 10 minutes
Cooking time: 12 minutes
Servings: 4
Ingredients:

- 1 zucchini, thinly sliced
- A pinch of sea salt
- Black pepper to taste
- 1 tsp. thyme, dried
- 1 egg
- 1 tsp. garlic powder
- 1 cup almond flour

Directions:

1. In a bowl, whisk the egg with a pinch of salt.
2. Put the flour in another bowl and mix it with thyme, black pepper, and garlic powder.
3. Dredge zucchini slices in the egg mix and then in flour.
4. Arrange chips on a lined baking sheet, place in the oven at 450°F and bake for 6 minutes on each side,
5. Serve the zucchini chips as a snack. Enjoy.

Nutrition:

- Calories: 106
- Fat: 8.2g
- Protein: 5.1g

91. Pepperoni Bites

Preparation time: 5 minutes
Cooking time: 10 minutes
Servings: 24 pieces
Ingredients:

- ⅓ cup tomatoes, chopped
- ½ cup bell peppers, mixed and chopped
- 24 pepperoni slices
- ½ cup tomato sauce
- 4 oz. almond cheese, cubed
- 2 tbsps. basil, chopped
- Black pepper to taste

Directions:

1. Divide pepperoni slices into a muffin tray.
2. Divide tomato and bell pepper pieces into the pepperoni cups.
3. Also divide the tomato sauce, basil, and almond cheese cubes, sprinkle black pepper at the end, place cups in the oven at 400°F, and bake for 10 minutes.
4. Arrange the pepperoni bites on a platter and serve.

Nutrition:

- Calories: 59
- Fat: 4.5g
- Protein: 2.5g

92. Beet Blast Smoothie

Preparation time: 5 minutes
Cooking time: 0 minutes
Servings: 1
Ingredients:

- 1½ cups unsweetened plant-based milk
- 1 Granny Smith apple, peeled, cored, and chopped
- 1 cup chopped frozen beets
- 1 cup frozen blueberries
- ½ cup frozen cherries
- ¼-inch fresh ginger root, peeled

Directions:

1. In a blender, combine all the ingredients and blend until smooth.
2. Serve immediately or store in the freezer in a resalable jar.

Nutrition:

- Calories: 324
- Fat: 5g
- Protein: 5g

93. Green Power Smoothie

Preparation time: 5 minutes
Cooking time: 0 minutes
Servings: 1
Ingredients:

- 3 cups fresh spinach
- 1½ cups frozen pineapple
- 1 cup unsweetened plant-based milk
- 1 cup fresh kale
- 1 Granny Smith apple, peeled, cored, and chopped
- ½ small avocado, pitted and peeled
- ½ tsp. spirulina
- 1 tbsp. hemp seeds

Directions:

1. In a blender, combine all the ingredients and blend until smooth.
2. Serve immediately or store in the freezer in a resalable jar.

Nutrition:

- Calories: 431
- Fat: 16g
- Protein: 13g

94. Tropical Bliss Smoothie

Preparation time: 5 minutes
Cooking time: 0 minutes
Servings: 1
Ingredients:

- 2 cups frozen pineapple
- 1 banana
- 1¼ cups unsweetened coconut milk
- ¼ cup frozen coconut pieces
- ½ tsp. ground flaxseed
- 1 tsp. hemp seeds

Directions:

1. In a blender, combine all the ingredients and blend until smooth.
2. Serve immediately or store in the freezer in a resalable jar.

Nutrition:

- Calories: 396
- Fat: 14g
- Protein: 6g

95. Very Berry Antioxidant Smoothie

Preparation time: 5 minutes
Cooking time: 0 minutes
Servings: 1
Ingredients:

- 1 banana
- 1¼ cups unsweetened plant-based milk
- ½ cup frozen strawberries
- ½ cup frozen blueberries
- ½ cup frozen raspberries
- 3 pitted Medjool dates
- 1 tbsp. hulled hemp seeds
- ½ tbsp. ground flaxseed
- 1 tsp. ground chia seeds

Directions:

1. In a blender, combine all the ingredients and blend until smooth.
2. Serve immediately or store in the freezer in a resalable jar.

Nutrition:

- Calories: 538
- Fat: 11g
- Protein: 10g

96. Easy Overnight Oats

Preparation time: 5 minutes, plus overnight
Cooking time: 0 minutes
Servings: 1
Ingredients:

- ½ cup rolled oats (check the label for gluten-free)
- ½ cup unsweetened plant-based milk
- 1 tbsp. nut butter
- ½ tbsp. cacao powder
- ½ tsp. hulled hemp hearts
- ½ tsp. maple syrup

Optional toppings:

- Dark chocolate chips
- Pecans
- Strawberries

Directions:

1. Combine all the ingredients in a Mason jar or reusable food storage container.
2. Stir together, seal the lid, and place in the refrigerator overnight.
3. When ready to eat, add your favorite toppings.

Nutrition:

- Calories: 347
- Fat: 14g
- Protein: 12g

97. Apple-Cinnamon Quinoa

Preparation time: 5 minutes
Cooking time: 5 minutes
Servings: 1
Ingredients:

- 1½ cups water
- 1½ cups diced Granny Smith apples
- ½ cup quinoa, rinsed
- 1 tsp. ground flaxseed
- ½ tsp. ground cinnamon

Optional toppings:

- Maple syrup
- Nuts and seeds
- Nut butter
- Fresh fruit
- Unsweetened plant-based milk

Directions:

1. In a medium pot over medium-high heat, combine the water, apples, quinoa, and flaxseed for 5 minutes, or until the water has been fully absorbed.
2. Transfer the quinoa mixture to a bowl and stir in the cinnamon.
3. Serve immediately as is or with your favorite toppings.

Nutrition:

- Calories: 456
- Fat: 7g
- Protein: 13g

98. Strawberry-Kiwi Chia Pudding

Preparation time: 5 minutes, plus 4 hours
Cooking time: 0 minutes
Servings: 2
Ingredients:

- 2 cups unsweetened coconut milk, divided
- 3 Medjool dates, pitted
- 1 tbsp. vanilla extract
- ½ cup chia seeds

Toppings:

- 2 kiwis, sliced
- 4 strawberries, sliced
- 2 tbsps. unsweetened coconut shreds
- 2 tbsps. sliced or chopped almonds

Directions:

1. In a food processor, blend ¾ cup of coconut milk, the dates, and vanilla.
2. Pour the blended mix into a large reusable container or Mason jar.
3. Add the remaining 1¼ cups of coconut milk and the chia seeds.
4. Cover the container and shake gently or stir to mix.
5. Store in the refrigerator overnight or for at least 4 hours, until the chia seeds absorb all the milk. (Optional: stir once or twice as it is setting to avoid clumps.)
6. When ready to eat, top the pudding with kiwi, strawberries, coconut, and almonds.
7. Store in the refrigerator for up to 5 days.

Nutrition:

- Calories: 783
- Fat: 38g
- Protein: 27g

99. Banana Protein Pancakes

Preparation time: 5 minutes
Cooking time: 15 minutes
Servings: 2
Ingredients:

- 1½ cups unsweetened plant-based milk
- 1 cup quick oats
- 1 banana
- ½ cup vital wheat gluten
- ½ cup whole wheat flour
- 2 tbsps. maple syrup
- 2 tsps. vanilla extract
- 1 tsp. pink Himalayan salt

Optional toppings:

- Sliced bananas
- Pecans
- Hulled hemp seeds
- Maple syrup

Directions:

1. In a food processor, combine all the ingredients except the optional toppings and mix until smooth.
2. Use a 1/4-cup measuring cup to pour 1/6 of the batter into a nonstick skillet over medium heat.
3. Once the edges of the pancake start to brown and bubble, flip and cook the other side.
4. Repeat with the remaining batter.
5. Serve immediately with your favorite toppings (if using) or store the pancakes in the refrigerator in a sealed container for up to 3 days.

Nutrition:

- Calories: 546
- Fat: 6g
- Protein: 36g

100. Blueberry Scones

Preparation time: 5 minutes, plus 20 minutes to freeze
Cooking time: 25 minutes
Servings: 6
Ingredients:

- 2 cups whole wheat flour
- ½ cup coconut sugar
- 2½ tsps. baking powder
- ½ tsp. pink Himalayan salt
- ½ cup unsweetened applesauce
- 3 tbsps. aquafaba (the liquid from a can of chickpeas)
- 2½ tsps. vanilla extract
- ⅓ cup chopped almonds
- 1 cup fresh blueberries

Directions:

1. Preheat the oven to 400°F.
2. In a large bowl, mix the flour, coconut sugar, baking powder, and salt. Add the applesauce, aquafaba, and vanilla and mix the dough together by hand. Gently stir in the almonds and blueberries.
3. Line an 8-inch square baking pan with parchment paper and spread the dough evenly in the pan.
4. Freeze the dough for 20 minutes.
5. Bake for 25 minutes, or until light brown. Once cooled, cut into 6 scones.
6. Store at room temperature in a covered container for up to 5 days.

Nutrition:

- Calories: 265
- Fat: 3g
- Protein: 5g

101. Cinnamon French Toast

Preparation time: 5 minutes
Cooking time: 10 minutes
Servings: 2
Ingredients:

- 1 cup unsweetened plant-based milk
- ¾ cup firm tofu
- ½ tsp. vanilla extract
- ½ tsp. ground cinnamon
- ¼ tsp. ground flaxseed
- 4 slices thick whole wheat bread

Directions:

1. In a blender, blend the milk, tofu, vanilla, cinnamon, and flaxseed until smooth.
2. Pour the mixture into a wide bowl.
3. Dip the bread slices into the mixture until evenly coated on both sides.
4. In a medium nonstick pan over medium heat, cook the bread slices, flipping when the bottom is light brown. Flip again, if needed.

Nutrition:

- Calories: 642
- Fat: 20g
- Protein: 31g

Conclusion

In anything new that we try, there is a chance that we may fall off track. Fasting or following a new diet plan is no different. The focus should not be on the fact that you fell off but on how you decide to come back and approach it again. You need not give up altogether if you have a day or two where you did not accomplish your full fast. You just need to re-examine your plan and approach it differently. Maybe your fasting period was too long for your first try. Maybe your fasting and eating windows did not match up with your sleep-wake cycle as well as they could have. Any of these factors can be adjusted to better suit your lifestyle needs and make fasting or a specific diet work for you. Being able to be flexible with yourself is something that trying a new diet regimen like this can teach you. With the human body, there is never a right or a wrong way to approach anything; there is only a multitude of different ways and some that will be better for your specific body and mind than others. Being open to trying different variations and adjusting your plan as you go can be the difference between success and the decision to give up.

If you fall off track, scale your plan back a little bit and try it again. If you are worried that you are not doing enough, begin with the scaled-back plan, and get used to this first, you can always increase your fasting times later on once you know you are completely comfortable with a shorter fasting time.

If this guidebook has taught you anything, the hope is that it has taught you how many variables are involved when it comes to health and wellness. This guidebook aimed to share with you the plethora of options that are available to you when it comes to intermittent fasting for women over 50.

Think back on the many options that were laid out for you in this guidebook involving diet options and specific foods that can induce autophagy in the brain. It is your job now to decide which of these foods or supplements to include in your life and to practice a sort of trial and error, noting which ones make you feel great and which ones you prefer to go without. With all of this information, you can decide which ways fit best with your specific lifestyle and your preferences.

As you take all of this information forth with you, it may seem overwhelming to begin applying this to your own life. Remember, life is a process, and you do not need to expect perfection from yourself. By taking the steps to read this guidebook, you are already on your way to changing your life. IF you fall off of the diet and you need inspiration, come back and review this guidebook and remind yourself why you wanted to begin it in the first place.

Made in the USA
Monee, IL
03 September 2021